Aging Bravely

(Shut Up and Stop Your Whining!)

Dana Racinskas

THIS BOOK BELONGS TO:

_____

DEDICATION

This book is dedicated to my two moms: Adele, my mother, and Irene, my mother-in-law. Through war and famine and journeying to a foreign land to provide better lives for their children, they somehow maintained resolute bravery and lust for life. Theirs were truly lives well-lived.

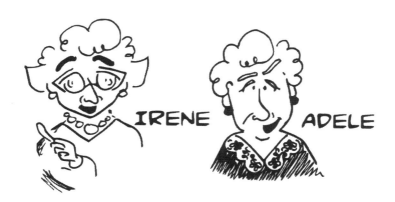

IRENE   ADELE

Old age is no place for sissies.

Bette Davis

Spirit is ageless.

Unknown

CONTENTS

ACKNOWLEDGMENTS

This book wouldn't be in your hands right now if it weren't for the loving support of my family. The love and companionship my husband provides has sustained me for more than thirty years. The joy and pride my children and grandchild provide inspires me to age bravely for them.

Thanks to my son, Jon Racinskas, who has graciously and patiently helped me put to paper the words that have been in my heart for many years.

Thanks to our illustrator, Rachel Koskelin, who somehow found a way to bring the spirit of "the two moms" to these pages.

Finally, thanks to our editor, Amanda Johnson, whose meticulous attention to detail drove us crazy. (There, their, they're…got it.)

1 AGING BRAVELY

Many things in life are easy because we know how to do them instinctively. Take breathing for example; if it weren't an autonomic function requiring absolutely no action on our part, how many of us would have forgotten to breathe before we left the house this morning? *Let's see – I've got my coffee, keys, and glasses, so why do I feel like I'm forgetting something? Oh yeah! Air!*

Getting older isn't really one of those instinctual things. While it's true that the changes at the cellular, tissue, and organ levels associated with aging are, to a large extent, completely out of our control, we must all *learn* how to grow old.

At my current "day job," I am on call twenty-four hours a day as the Nurse Practitioner for a number of nursing homes in the Dallas area. When you've worked as long as I have in geriatrics -- which is longer than I'd care to say – you can say with some certainty that you've "seen it all". In fact you've seen it all for so long that even the super crazy stuff has become commonplace. But this book isn't a collection of a nurse's "war stories". It is a warning to all of you.

No matter how many times I see it, this manages to break my heart every time: many seniors have absolutely no idea how to live their "golden years;" they stick with the "default settings," meaning they only see aging as a physical process and not as a phase of life. Consequently, their aging becomes an increasing burden on both them and their loved ones.

But I don't blame them. How could I? Nothing really prepares us for this—any of us. Both seniors and their adult children are forced to tread an unfamiliar path. The roles gradually reverse and the parents who taught those children to walk and talk now need guidance themselves.

Think about the last time you were in a bookstore.[1] How many books did you see on child development? There are thousands and thousands of them on those shelves, far too many to read in a single lifetime.[2]

You can also watch child development videos, attend special classes and even consult one-on-one with experts. These are all wonderful tools to help

---

[1] At the time of this writing, bookstores still existed.

[2] Did you know Dr. Spock's *Baby and Child Care* is the second-best-selling book of all time, surpassed only by the Bible?

guide you through times of significant physical and emotional changes in your child.

But what about your 72 year-old mother? Can you point me to the aisle for "senior *development*" books? Where are the videos, special classes, and consultations to help guide you through the time of significant physical and emotional changes in your parent? For the most part, these do not exist.

So, why, when we've put some much effort into understanding one phase of human development, do we make so little effort to understand another? I believe that when it comes to seniors, we, as a society, fail to distinguish between *development* and *decline.*

Think about it; when your three year-old throws a tantrum because you won't buy her an ice cream, do you take it personally? Hopefully not. You realize, if only subconsciously, that this is normal for a child in this particular phase of development. So why, then, do we not offer seniors the same courtesy? Why do we write off certain behaviors as merely a decline in their faculties? Why are we impatient with them? Are they not entering a new stage of development themselves? Their bodies and minds are changing once again— whether they realize it or not. Their relationships are changing as well. The "kids" have become the adults—most likely with children of their own— who must now adjust to helping guide those who patiently taught and guided them. Welcome to the "Sandwich Generation."

As we explore the issues inherent in this stage of life, there is one thing to always bear in mind: Seniors have never been elderly before, so this is uncharted territory for them too. We are all heading in the same direction, and none of us has a map.

The purpose of this book is to help both seniors and their adult children "take the bull by the horns" by confronting certain realities of aging. This will allow seniors to move forward, free of fear and frustration, and to live their lives to their fullest potential – to *age bravely*.

My goal is to help you fully understand the issues and inspire you to *actively* and *fearlessly* address them—to make a plan for dealing with the senior transition and stick with it. For the adult offspring reading this book, I would urge you to, as you read, apply these lessons to your life as well. Talk with your own kids about these things; you're not just learning how to help your elderly parent, but also yourself, your spouse, and your kids. You will be in a similar position sooner than you think.

This certainly won't be easy, but if these issues aren't addressed, if you don't talk about them

---

RANDOM FACT: IN EUREKA, NEVADA, IT IS ILLEGAL FOR MEN WHO HAVE MUSTACHES TO KISS WOMEN.

because you perceive them as awkward or even morbid, *you are in for a world of hurt*. I've seen these issues tear families apart so often that, tragically, it has become commonplace for me. Do us both a favor and don't become just another one of those stories.

By purchasing this book, you've taken a critical first step – desiring to educate yourself on this stage of life. I will help you take the next steps – talking about and acting on what you've learned.

First, a couple quick notes on the format of this book: At the end of each chapter is a list of "Talking Points." These are there to be used as "crib notes," quick reference for the most important points you will need to address in your elder parent/ adult child dialogues. Use them. Also, the footnotes on several of these pages contain factoids, opinions, and references. They're worth reading, too.

This book is designed to be written in, so take lots of notes. They'll be really helpful when you begin formulating your plan.

If you get lost in the reading or just need someone to talk to, you can always reach me on the Facebook page: Facebook.com/AgingBravely. We're in this together.

Ready to get "Brave?" Then, let's get started!

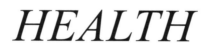

HEALTH

2 THE ADVANCE DIRECTIVE

March 31, 2005: The sad announcement the world has been waiting for finally comes: After an epic seven-year legal battle, Terri Schiavo has died. Newscasters around the globe remark how easily this whole ordeal could have been avoided had Schiavo only recorded an advance directive.

An advance directive is a legal document that helps to ensure your wishes regarding various medical treatments are followed in the event you become unable to make your own decisions.

In many states, the term "advance directive" is actually referring to two individual directives: a "proxy directive" and an "instruction directive." It is often your decision whether to have both kinds or just one.[3] Each directive addresses a specific, but equally important, role in protecting your wishes

---

RANDOM FACT: FIRST COUSINS MAY MARRY IN UTAH, BUT ONLY AFTER THEY'RE 65 YEARS OLD.

[3] The specific requirements for the content of an Advance Directive vary by state, so be sure to do the research. You can find all 50 states here: http://www.caringinfo.org/i4a/pages/index.cfm?pageid=3289

pertaining to your healthcare, and I implore you to prepare both.

DURABLE HEALTHCARE POWER OF ATTORNEY (aka "Proxy Directive")
Durable Healthcare Power of Attorney is a document in which you appoint a trusted friend or family member to make important healthcare decisions for you in the event you become unable to make them yourself. This document goes into effect whether your inability to make healthcare decisions is temporary because of an accident or permanent because of a disease. The person you appoint is known as your "healthcare representative" and he is responsible for making the same decisions you would have made under the circumstances. If he is unable to determine what you would want in a specific situation, he is to base his decision on what he thinks is in your best interest.

THE LIVING WILL (aka "Instruction Directive")
A living will is a document you use to let your doctor and family know what you want them to do in medical situations where life-sustaining treatment must be considered and you're not coherent enough to tell them yourself. You can also talk about your personal beliefs and values if they affect such decisions. This additional document is really helpful in situations not specifically covered by your

advance directive.[4]

The Schiavo story marked the first time many Americans had heard of an advance directive; the fear of ending up like her, with their families being torn apart while the world watches, caused many of them to scramble to record their own end-of-life wishes. But this was not, however, a lesson learned. In fact, recent polls show that less than 25% of Americans have created an advance directive, which is about the same number as before the Schiavo debacle. Nothing has changed.

Let's now take a look at a couple of reasons *why* many people don't have an advance directive prepared:

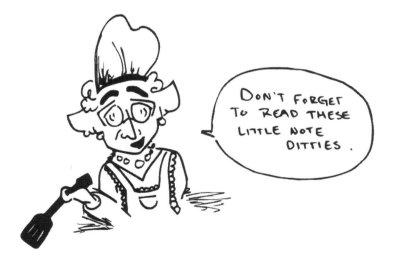

---

[4] From the State of New Jersey Department of Health

- *I don't want to be denied healthcare simply because I have an advance directive.* You may not believe it, but this is one of the most common reasons people don't have an advance directive—they truly believe healthcare will be withheld from them if they have one. What really gets me is that these people fail to see the ridiculousness of this assumption. A surgeon will *not* shrug off the Hippocratic Oath and deny you the gallstone surgery you so desperately need simply because you may not share their opinion on life-sustaining measures (unless malpractice lawyers suddenly disappeared).

- *I don't want my family to have to "pull the plug." I want them to have options.* This is a misconception very similar to the healthcare denial myth; in reality, your living will can demand every life-sustaining measure under the sun.

None of us would say we want someone else to determine how we die, and yet without an advance directive, without recording our end-of-life wishes, this is essentially what we are asking someone else to do. You lived your life on your terms, so why not see that through to the end?

RANDOM FACT: A 2008 MARKET STUDY IN YOGA JOURNAL REPORTS THAT SOME 16 MILLION AMERICANS PRACTICE YOGA AND SPEND $5.7 BILLION A YEAR ON GEAR.

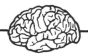

DID YOU KNOW?

The family of Terri Schiavo endured 14 appeals and numerous motions, petitions and hearings in Florida courts, five suits in federal district court, Florida legislation struck down by the Supreme Court of Florida, federal legislation (the "Palm Sunday Compromise", and four denials of certiorari from the Supreme Court of the United States before they were able to say their final goodbyes.

All of this could have been avoided had she completed an advance directive.

HOW TO COMPLETE AN ADVANCE DIRECTIVE

Before we begin, I'd like to give you a bit of fair warning: Some of this is pretty complicated stuff. However, if you run across a term or phrase you don't understand, don't sweat it. I'll break the whole thing down into easily digestible pieces later in the chapter. Ready to jump in?

The next few pages contain a great example of an advance directive which you can actually use in a number of states.[5] Read each section carefully. Before you fill out the form, *talk to the person you want to name as having Durable Health Care Power of Attorney, to make sure that he/she understands your wishes and is willing to take on this responsibility.* (Seriously, don't just spring this kind of thing on a person.) Write your initials in the blank spaces next to the choices you want to make. Write your initials only beside the choices you want under Parts 1, 2 and 3 of this form. Your advance directive should be valid for whichever part(s) you fill in, as long as it is properly signed.

Add any special instructions in the blank spaces provided. You can write additional comments on a separate sheet of paper, but you should make a note on this form that there are additional pages you wish to be included with your advance directive.

---

[5] Again, be sure to check the requirements of your state.

Sign the form and have it witnessed. Give copies to your lawyer, your doctor, your nurse, the person you name to make your medical decisions for you (power of attorney or "POA"), people in your family, and anyone else who might be involved in your care. Discuss your advance directive with them all,[6] and update them about any changes.

---

[6] **An important note:** You can change this document at any time, but make sure that the people who need to have it only have one version in their possession. If you give them a new draft, collect the old one.

MY ADVANCE DIRECTIVE

I,_____,
write this document as a directive regarding my
medical care.

**In the following sections, put the initials of your
name in the blank spaces by the choices you
want.**

PART 1. My Durable Power of Attorney for Health Care

_____ **I appoint this person to make decisions
about my medical care if there ever comes a time
when I cannot make those decisions myself. I
want the person I have appointed, my doctors,
my family, and others to be guided by the
decisions I have made in the parts of the form
that follow.**

Name:_____

Home telephone: _____

Work telephone: _____

Address:

_____

_____

If the person above cannot or will not make decisions for me, I appoint this person:

Name: _____

Home telephone: _____

Work telephone: _____

Address:

_____

_____

_____ **I have not appointed anyone to make health care decisions for me in this or any other document.**

PART 2. My Living Will

These are my wishes for my future medical care if there ever comes a time when I can't make these decisions for myself.

A. These are my wishes if I have a terminal condition:

Life-sustaining treatments

_____ I do not want life-sustaining treatment (including CPR) started. If life-sustaining treatments are started, I want them stopped.

_____ I want the life-sustaining treatments that my doctors think are best for me.

_____ Other wishes

_____

_____

Artificial nutrition and hydration

_____ I do not want artificial nutrition and hydration started if they would be the main treatments keeping me alive. If artificial nutrition and hydration are started, I want them stopped.

_____ I want artificial nutrition and hydration even if they are the main treatments keeping me alive.

_____ Other wishes

_____

_____

Comfort care

_____ I want to be kept as comfortable and free of pain as possible, even if such care prolongs my dying or shortens my life.

_____ Other wishes

_____

_____

B. These are my wishes if I am ever in a persistent vegetative state:

Life-sustaining treatments

_____ I do not want life-sustaining treatments (including CPR) started. If life-sustaining treatments are started, I want them stopped.

_____ I want the life-sustaining treatments that my doctors think are best for me.

_____ Other wishes

_____

_____

Artificial nutrition and hydration

_____ I do not want artificial nutrition and hydration started if they would be the main treatments keeping me alive. If artificial nutrition and hydration are started, I want them stopped.

_____ I want artificial nutrition and hydration even if they are the main treatments keeping me alive.

_____ Other wishes

_____

_____

Comfort care

_____ I want to be kept as comfortable and free of pain as possible, even if such care prolongs my dying or shortens my life.

_____ Other wishes

_____

_____

C. Other directions

You have the right to be involved in all decisions about your medical care, even those not dealing with terminal conditions or persistent vegetative states. If you have wishes not covered in other parts of this document, please indicate them below.

_____

_____

_____

_____

_____

_____

PART 3. Other Wishes

A. Organ donation

_____ I do not wish to donate any of my organs or tissues.

_____ I want to donate all of my organs and tissues.

_____ I only want to donate these organs and tissues:

_____

_____ Other wishes

_____

_____

B. Autopsy

_____ I do not want an autopsy.

_____ I agree to an autopsy if my doctors wish it.

_____ Other wishes

_____

_____

C. Other statements about your medical care

If you wish to say more about any of the choices you have made or if you have any other statements to make about your medical care, you may do so on a separate piece of paper. If you do so, put here the number of pages you are adding: _____

<u>PART 4. Signatures</u>

You and two witnesses must sign this document before it will be legal.

A. Your signature

By my signature below, I show that I understand the purpose and the effect of this document.

Signature

_____

Date _____

Address

_____

_____

B. Your witnesses' signatures

I believe the person who has signed this advance directive to be of sound mind, that he/she signed or acknowledged this advance directive in my presence, and that he/she appears not to be acting under pressure, duress, fraud, or undue influence. I am not related to the person making this advance directive by blood, marriage, or adoption nor, to the best of my knowledge, am I named in his/her will. I am not the person appointed in this advance directive. I am not a health care provider or an employee of a health care provider who is now, or has been in the past, responsible for the care of the person making this advance directive.

Witness #1

Signature

_____

Date _____

Address

_____

_____

Witness #2

Signature

_____

Date _____

Address

_____

_____

(CUT OUT & FILE YOUR WITH YOUR WILL)

That document was a little daunting, right? There are a bunch of terms in there I'll bet you haven't seen before, so I'm going to break it down for you, piece-by-piece, to make sure you understand what it is you've just read.

Part 1: Durable Health Care Power of Attorney Despite the name, this will have absolutely nothing to do with attorneys (insert sigh of relief). What it does is establish who speaks for you when you can't speak for yourself. This should be someone you trust completely, as there may come a time when this person will have to make significant choices for you. His agency, or authority to act on your behalf, becomes effective at any point when you may be deemed legally incompetent (coma, vegetative state, etc.). He will have the authority to handle your hospital discharge, authorize treatments, and even have your teeth cleaned.

Part 2: The Living Will This part usually provides specific instructions about the course of treatment that is to be followed by health care providers; it only becomes effective when you've become unable to provide informed consent or refusal due to some sort of incapacitation.

Your living will can be as general or specific as you like. Really specific living wills may include information regarding your position on such things as a DNR Order ("Do Not Resuscitate" – discussed at length in Chapter 3), analgesia (pain relief), food/

water, and the use of ventilators or CPR.

Note: Parts 1 and 2 probably seem very similar, but the distinction between them is significant and of vital importance. Basically, the living will focuses on end-of-life decisions. It's concerned with medical treatments when there's no hope of recovery. However, Durable Health Care Power of Attorney (DHCPOA) is much broader. It gives the assigned person, be it an adult child or trusted friend, the power to make decisions on your parent's behalf at a time when he or she is unable to (becomes legally incompetent).

The standards are these: The living will becomes effective when a doctor determines the condition to be terminal. DHCPOA becomes effective when the person is incapable of making decisions.

Part 3 is the miscellaneous part of our example, often called "My Particular Wishes." You can use it to spell out what you want done with your body after you're no longer using it. You can choose to be an organ donor here (it's a nice thing to do – help save a life, even after death). You can also choose whether or not you want an autopsy performed on your body. This is also where you could put your Dementia Clause (discussed in the

---

RANDOM FACT: THE PROTEIN THAT KEEPS A BABY'S SKULL FROM FUSING IS CALLED "NOGGIN".

next chapter). If you have any other requirements, put them here.

Part 4 is one of the most important parts - if you don't sign your advance directive, it can't be executed. Here's why this is so important: If you do not have a signed advance directive in place and you somehow lose the ability to make informed decisions about your treatment (i.e. you're deemed "legally incompetent"), your family will have to go through the arduous task of going to court to seek guardianship over you.

The petition for guardianship is a public proceeding, with which always comes the possibility that some "dirty laundry" may be aired for one and all to see. The court will be looking out for your best interest and will heavily scrutinize any individual(s) seeking guardianship. As with many legal proceedings, this may drag on for quite a while—it took seven years for the Schiavos to resolve the matter.

Bottom line: if you don't assign someone to make the decisions for you when you're not able to, someone else *will*. If you want to be involved in the process, make that decision *now.*

RANDOM FACT: ALL DOGS CAN BE TRACED BACK 40 MILLION YEARS AGO TO A WEASEL-LIKE ANIMAL CALLED THE MIACIS, WHICH DWELLED IN TREES AND DENS.

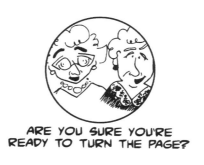

THE TALKING POINTS

This won't be an easy conversation to have. Of all the issues to talk about in this book, this one is the one your parent is likely to see as "morbid." It's easy to see why—it deals with what will happen when someone can't make important decisions for him or herself. This makes people uneasy because they perceive it as losing control, and it's really important that you stress that an advance directive does *exactly the opposite*. This document *gives* people control, even when they can't speak for themselves.

- Stroke or coma could suddenly leave you voiceless and force your family to guess as to what you would want.
- We need to know what you want in order to make sure you get it.
- We need to know *who* you want to speak for you when you can no longer speak for yourself.
- If you don't do this, everything you've tried to protect (dignity, independence, and legacy) is at great risk.
- Set a deadline for getting this done and mark it on your calendar. Peace of mind awaits you.
- Face these facts bravely.

3 THE DEMENTIA CLAUSE

The advance directive we just discussed is vitally important, but there is a significant limitation: Most advance directives only go into effect when a person is unable to make health care decisions and is either "permanently unconscious" or "terminally ill." There is usually no provision that applies to a situation in which a person suffers from severe dementia, but is neither unconscious nor dying. In short, if at some point your body is still healthy but your mind can no longer make informed decisions regarding your welfare, a dementia clause in your advance directive will neutralize potential conflicts with your intended course of care.

What is "dementia" and why should I be worried about it? Dementia is defined as a decline of reasoning, memory, and cognitive function. We used to call it "senility" and considered it a normal part of aging. As our knowledge of brain function progressed, the medical community ceased using the term "senility" and started calling it "dementia," which more accurately described the cognitive degeneration we were witnessing. We stopped thinking about it in a folksy sort of way, like that's just what happens to old people ("Granny's getting senile, tee hee."), and started seeing it as something far more serious. Now we know dementia is *not* a normal part of aging. We now see it for what it is: It's a disease, and it's running rampant.

How big of a problem is this? There are 4-5 million people in America over the age of 65 who are currently afflicted with some degree of dementia, and that number is only increasing as the "Baby Boomers" get on in age. According to the World Health Organization, the current cost for treating dementia in the U.S. is $604 billion and rising.

"/> At present, about 1% of the world's population aged 60 to 64 is afflicted with dementia, and one person is diagnosed every *four seconds*. From ages 65 to 84, that number doubles every five years. By age 85, the number skyrockets to somewhere between 30 and 50% of the population.

Those numbers should scare you. Up to half of our senior population may be suffering from some form of dementia, and only a small part of that number have a plan to deal with it. (More on that

---

"/)RANDOM FACT: IN TRURO, MISSISSIPPI, A MAN MUST PROVE HIMSELF WORTHY BEFORE GETTING MARRIED BY HUNTING AND KILLING EITHER SIX BLACKBIRDS OR THREE CROWS.

later.)

How is dementia related to Alzheimer's?
"Dementia" is a broad term that encompasses several diagnostic subcategories and levels of disability. Let's hit the basics—the two main categories are Alzheimer's and Non-Alzheimer's dementias.[7]

The Alzheimer's category is characterized predominantly by memory loss, accompanied by impairment in other cognitive (thinking) functions, such as language function (aphasia), skilled motor functions (apraxia), or perception, visual or other (agnosias)[8].

Non-Alzheimer dementias include the frontotemporal lobar degenerations, which generally are of two main types: One primarily affects speech, as in the primary progressive aphasia syndromes. The other is characterized primarily by changes in behavior, including apathy, disinhibition, personality change, and what is called executive function (e.g., planning ahead and organizational ability). In both of these types of dementia, memory loss is relatively mild, if present, until later in the course of the disease.

---

[7] From alz.org, the Alzheimer's Association's online wealth of knowledge.

[8] National Institute of Neurological Disorders Stroke. NINDS Dementia Information Page.

Other forms of dementia—including vascular disorders (multiple strokes), dementia with Lewy bodies, Parkinson's dementia, and normal pressure hydrocephalus—would be grouped among the non-Alzheimer disorders.

That was a lot of doctor-speak. Let's take a look at symptoms for which you should be keeping an eye out. Initially, dementia comes across as more a nuisance than a threat. You might find yourself having the same conversation over and over with your parent. You might spend more and more of your time on keys and glasses scavenger hunts. Then, things might get worse. The kitchen may flood due to forgotten faucets. Maybe you start to see more scorched pans and towels lying around the kitchen. From there, well, you get the picture.

I'm afraid I've got some more bad news for you—diagnosing dementia isn't an easy process. If your loved one's healthcare providers suspect dementia, they will first evaluate for chemical or organ troubles. Metabolic and diagnostic tests are performed to rule out treatable physical disorders.

If they don't find the answers there, the healthcare team will begin to administer tests for

---

RANDOM FACT: THE FIRST FILM EVER MADE IN HOLLYWOOD WAS D.W. GRIFFITH'S 1910 IN OLD CALIFORNIA, A BIOGRAPHIC MELODRAMA ABOUT A SPANISH MAIDEN (MARION LEONARD) WHO HAS AN ILLEGITIMATE SON WITH A MAN WHO LATER BECOMES GOVERNOR OF CALIFORNIA. IT WAS SHOT IN TWO DAYS.

cognitive function. They'll want to know how Dad's brain is working – how is he feeling? Is he disoriented, confused, or depressed? While not an exact science, these tests are standardized and research-proven, so they are very effective tools in diagnosis. They will first be administered to determine the cognitive degeneration and, later, to monitor the rate of progression.[9]

Is dementia treatable? I've always hated this answer, but it's necessary here: *it depends*. Almost all forms of dementia are *treatable*, but most of them are not *curable*. That's an important distinction to make because we have to manage our expectations here. Now, I'm not going to delve into detail on this one, as it's really a question for your doctor. Just know that there are treatment options available, and as our knowledge of this terrible disease continues to expand, so, too, will the options.

How would a dementia clause help us? The purpose of a dementia clause is to make the family and any medical staff aware of your parent's desired course of care, should Alzheimer's or some other form of dementia cause them to lose the ability to make those important decisions for themselves. The advance directive doesn't usually cover this, and as a consequence, they could cause loved ones sleepless nights spent wondering what your parent

---

[9] For examples of the tests administered, see the end of this chapter.

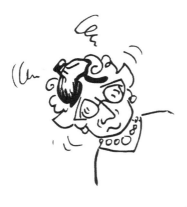

would want them to do. This is your opportunity to help them out. Remember those scary statistics we looked at earlier? There's a very real possibility that your parent could join that number. Give your family a break and address the topic now. Let them know what your parent wants by adding a dementia clause to their advance directive.

How do I address the dementia clause in my advance directive? Just sign and date the form on the next page and include it with the "My Particular Wishes" section in your advance directive or living will.[10]

---

[10] From compassionandchoices.org

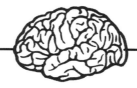

DID YOU KNOW?

The common causes of dementia:
-Degenerative neurological diseases, such as Alzheimer's, frontotemporal lobar degenerations, dementia with Lewy bodies, Parkinson's, and Huntington's
-Vascular disorders, such as multi-infarct dementia, which is caused by multiple strokes in the brain
-Infections that affect the central nervous system, such as HIV dementia complex and Creutzfeldt-Jakob disease

MY DEMENTIA CLAUSE

If I am unconscious and it is unlikely that I will ever become conscious again, I would like my wishes regarding specific life-sustaining treatments, as indicated on the attached document entitled "My Particular Wishes" to be followed.

If I remain conscious but have a progressive illness that will be fatal and the illness is in an advanced stage, and I am consistently and permanently unable to communicate, swallow food and water safely, care for myself, and recognize my family and other people, and it is very unlikely that my condition will substantially improve, I would like my wishes regarding specific life-sustaining treatments, as indicated on the attached document entitled "My Particular Wishes" to be followed. If I am unable to feed myself while in this condition I do / do not (circle one) want to be fed.

I hereby incorporate this provision in to my durable power of attorney for health care, living will, and any other previously executed advance directive for health care decisions.

Signature: _____

Date: _____

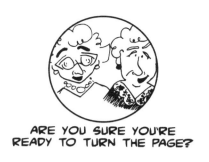

ARE YOU SURE YOU'RE
READY TO TURN THE PAGE?

THE TALKING POINTS

Here are the items you should be sure to cover in your discussion about a dementia clause:

- Reiterate who has been assigned Durable Healthcare Power of Attorney—this is super important; this person will have to make healthcare choices for them if they didn't already lay those out in their living will or advance directive.
- Talk about the statistics to emphasize the realness of the possibility; you need to be frank and honest. Talk about any fears you may have, for them, the family, and yourself.
- Examine the advance directive to see if you've addressed what happens in the event of the onset of advanced dementia.
- If it's not addressed, talk about what the family should do when they can no longer make those decisions for themselves.
- Emphasize that there may come a time when their unintentional actions may make you sad, but that they should know that the

35

family knows it's part of the disease – it's nothing personal.

- Be sure to let them know that you will always love them, even if they can no longer recognize your face.

Examples of Cognitive Testing

These tests have been provided by the Alzheimer's Association (alz.org) to healthcare professionals for the purpose of identifying patients who need more thorough evaluation. All of these tests are relatively free of influence by educational level, so it doesn't matter if the patient has a GED or a PhD, the results will be the same.

1. A three-word delayed recall exercise

- Tell your patient to remember three words.

- Give three common nouns, such as horse, pencil, and rose; ask the patient to repeat them.

- About five minutes later, ask the patient to recall the three words.

    - Individuals without impairment should be able to remember all three words, especially with such prompts as, "The first word was the name of an animal."

    - Remembering only one or two words indicates a need for further evaluation.

2. The "mini-cog" test, combining three-word

recall with clock-drawing

- Give three simple nouns and ask the patient to repeat them.

- Ask the patient to draw the face of a clock on a sheet of paper, showing the time as 10 minutes past 11.

- After the clock has been drawn, ask the patient to repeat the three words.

  - Patients who remember all three words have no dementia.

  - Patients who remember none of the words should receive further evaluation.

  - If the patient remembers one or two words, the physician should refer to the score on the clock drawing to help interpret this result.
    - normal clock = non-demented

- abnormal clock = further evaluation needed

  ○ Patients who recall all three words but have a problem with the clock may also require further evaluation.

More about clock-drawing and scoring

- When stating the time to be shown on the clock, don't refer to the "hands" of the clock – that's prompting. Rather, say "Show the time as 10 past 11."

  ○ "10 past 11" tests the ability to translate "10 past" into the right numerical value.

  ○ It also requires the use of both halves of the clock face.

- There are several scoring systems. A simple one is based on four points, with a lower score suggesting further evaluation.

  ○ One point is given for drawing a closed circle. Some clinicians prefer to give patients a pre-drawn circle, so that any accidental distortions in shape do not affect the placement of the numbers.

- One point is awarded for including the 12 correct numbers.

- One point is given for putting the numbers in the correct position.

- One point is awarded for drawing the hands to show the correct time. The degree of difficulty in producing a correct time may be factored into the score.

3. Coin-counting exercise

- Ask your patient, "If I give you a nickel, a quarter, a dime, and a penny, how much money have I given you?"

- When you avoid naming the coins in ascending or descending order of value, this task calls upon comprehension, working (or task completion) memory, planning, and calculating skills.

Inability to arrive at the correct total of 41 cents may indicate a need for further evaluation.[11]

---

[11] See? Evaluating dementia actually involves a scientific approach and not just family members sitting around the table pondering the age-old question "just how crazy *is* the old bat?"

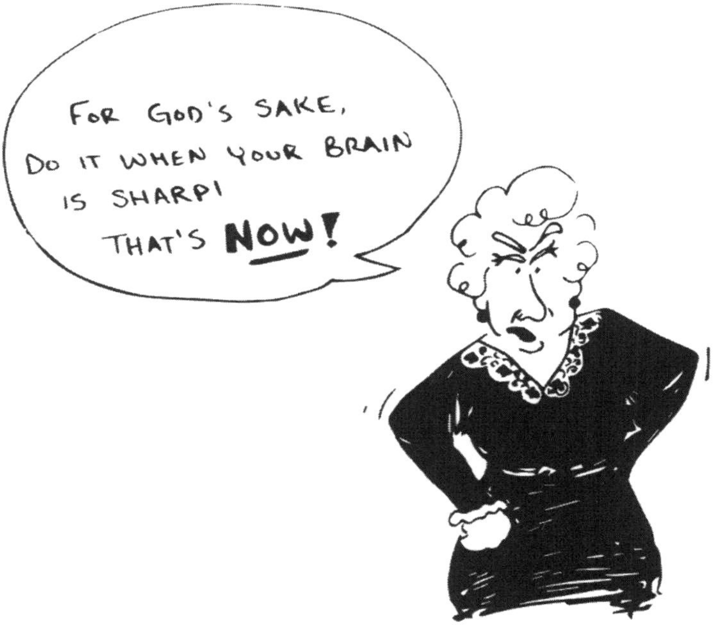
FOR GOD'S SAKE,
DO IT WHEN YOUR BRAIN
IS SHARP!
THAT'S NOW!

4 THE "DO NOT RESUSCITATE" (DNR)/ CARDIOPULMONARY RESUSCITATION (CPR) DEBATE

This will be one of the most awkward things we need discuss. It's awkward because you guys will have to consider the pros and cons of death. Confronting the DNR/CPR debate forces you to ask the question – *Do I want to go on living at any cost by using all that medical technology has to offer, or do I want to let nature decide when I go?*

What is a DNR Order (aka "No Code")? It's three simple letters written on a patient's chart, but it means a lot. Those letters let all the doctors and nurses in the hospital, or responding EMTs, know that if your parent's heart stops beating or they stop breathing, medical professionals shouldn't try to revive them. Essentially, the DNR relieves them of their duty to resuscitate – it says to the world that when their body says it's time to go, they just want to go. No interference. No pounding on their chest. No machines forcing air into their lungs. They just want to give their body what it wants – release.

So, why would anyone want a DNR? Let's take a realistic look at resuscitation.: Some of my patients can't seem to wrap their heads around the fact that the defibrillator is *not* a time machine. Hitting your body with enough voltage to light up Des Moines can't magically undo decades of degeneration—it can only prolong the inevitable. If your body is too worn out to go on, it will let you know. Defibrillation only confuses it momentarily. Your body will figure this out and restart the shut-down process. Of that, you can be absolutely sure.

If you're still not decided, here's another fact to consider: You most likely won't survive the hospital's resuscitation efforts. With all that drama and expense comes a *1-in-10* shot at making it. Also, as you get older, those odds get even worse. For some people, it's still worth a shot, but I doubt even Wall Street would take those odds!

Despite these facts, many people refuse a DNR —some for ridiculous reasons. There's a popular myth that if someone has a DNR, he or she will have healthcare withheld.

RANDOM FACT: THE MOST EXPENSIVE SWIMSUIT IN THE WORLD IS A BIKINI THAT IS WORTH $30 MILLION DOLLARS. DESIGNED BY SUSAN ROSEN AND STEINMETZ DIAMONDS, THE BIKINI IS MAD

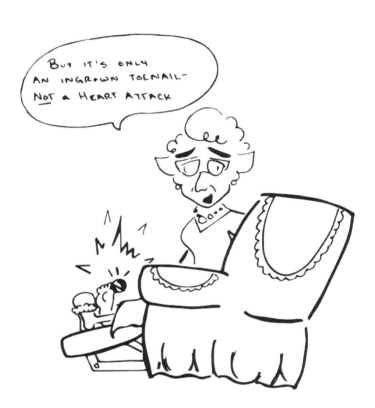

In reality, a DNR only addresses situations where someone is in a limited-life condition and doesn't wish to be artificially kept alive. It will *not* lead to their doctor refusing to help them if they go in for gallstones. In fact, if their heart stops in surgery for those gallstones, the doctors will attempt to restart it. If those efforts fail, the DNR "kicks in" and they won't put the patient on a ventilator just to keep them breathing.

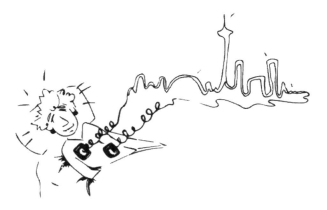

Another popular reason for refusing a DNR is simple fear. As human beings, we're wired to fight for survival. It is our instinct to do whatever we have to do to stay alive, and that's okay. However, sometimes we have to favor quality of life over quantity. Say you are successfully resuscitated, only to find yourself in a persistent vegetative state - you really don't want me to go into detail of what happens to your body while you lie there in that bed in essence dead to the world all because you couldn't get over your survival instinct. Let me just say, it's actually pretty gross. Yes, you are technically alive, but here's how you--a once proud person--may spend the those few days resuscitation just bought you: motionless in a bed, curled up in the fetal position in diapers, with a respirator doing your breathing and a tube pumping nutrition into your gut.

One of the things that people who refuse a DNR Order may not fully realize is the impact this will have on their family. The odds of an elderly patient surviving the resuscitation efforts is *beyond* slim. If the ER takes drastic measures to resuscitate, and that resuscitation fails, the body is often left the way it was when the patient passed. When the family is called in for their goodbyes, the body of their loved one is sometimes left bloody, naked, and bruised. This horrible sight could be someone's final memory of their loved one.[12]

With a DNR "No CPR" Order, the hospital staff knows that the patient wishes to be as comfortable as possible while nature takes its course. Theirs will be a death with dignity – clothed and with their loved ones in quiet attendance.

One more thing to consider before I conclude

---

[12] This actually happened to a friend of mine!

this chapter: Legacy is really important here. We will live and we will die, but what we do and say in between those two events can live on indefinitely.

When we are closer to the end of our lives than the beginning, our thoughts naturally turn to how we will be remembered. When making these decisions, your parent should give serious thought to how these decisions will impact how they are remembered.

Think about it: If you're ninety-two years old and in generally poor health, but feel compelled to require unlimited resuscitation, it won't matter how much your family loves you; they will come to see you as selfish. Why? Because every time you "code" in the middle of the night, they will get a phone call and have to rush to be by your side. I'm not going to candy-coat this: This gets *really* old *really* fast. After a while, they are forced to stop living their lives so they can be by your side for months. In the end, all of those cherished memories of a life well-lived could be tainted by the unspoken resentment the family built up while your parent struggled to find the courage to let go."/>

Despite your mother's words to the contrary, you're not special, especially in this regard: You will die just like everyone else does. The only thing

---

"/>RANDOM FACT: JUST TWO PERCENT OF THE WORLD'S POPULATION IS NATURALLY BLONDE.

you really have any influence over here is how you're remembered after. Making hard choices for yourself, instead of having others do it for you, helps to ensure you're remembered well.[13]

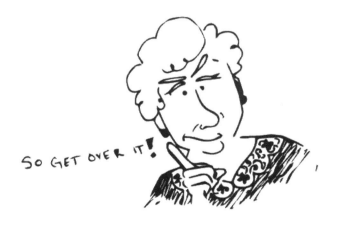

SO GET OVER IT!

---

[13] You can, however, make a requirement in the living will that there be no CPR administered. The will enable the doctor to write a DNR order.

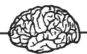

DID YOU KNOW?

Creating a DNR

Unlike the advance directive, you can't write up your own DNR. These are state-specific and must be signed by your doctor.

The specific structure of the DNR order will vary state-by-state, but the idea is universal.

Visit parentcarepro.com to find the form for your home state. Print one up and have it ready for the next doctor's appointment.

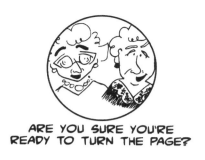

ARE YOU SURE YOU'RE
READY TO TURN THE PAGE?

THE TALKING POINTS

There's no way to have this conversation without both you and your parent coming off as at least a little bit selfish -- your parent because they may want to require resuscitation despite the futility, and you because you may prefer not to spend months or years of your life saying goodbye.

Still, it's a conversation that needs to be had. Be sure to talk about reasonable expectations in end-of-life issues.

- The older you are, the slimmer the chances of successful resuscitation.
- Your odds of surviving the ER's resuscitation efforts are about 10%. TV has skewed the public's perception on this – it won't bring you back.
- Even if it did, being resuscitated doesn't *fix* anything. In fact, resuscitation can *prolong* suffering.
- Seeking *quantity* over *quality* of years just doesn't make sense.

- It takes more guts to say "enough is enough" than to go on fighting a fight you cannot win; the house always wins in this case.
- Often, it's the adult children who don't want the DNR here. Remember: it's about *their* wishes.

5 ARTIFICIAL NUTRITION AND HYDRATION

Artificial nutrition and hydration (ANH) is a life-sustaining medical treatment whereby a mix of nutrients and fluids is forced into the body by placing a tube directly into the stomach, intestine, or a vein. When your loved one has reached a point where they can no longer eat and drink on their own, this healthcare option is available. But is it the right thing to do? In most cases, the answer is *no*. In fact, it's often the cruel thing to do; the risks inherent in the ANH process frequently offset the benefits.

Our instinct is to do whatever we can to prolong our loved one's life. Our love and gratitude for the role they played in our lives compels us to do all we can to "save" them. While a noble concept, this may not be the compassionate choice.

Your initial reaction to the proposition that anyone should deny a person food and water may be outrage, but I urge you to learn the facts and make an informed and objective decision together.

I have included a template for declaring your loved one's position on the matter at the end of this chapter. When they have reached their decision, have them fill it out and include it with their Advance Directive.

Here are the facts to consider:[14]

- Food and water are vital parts of the healing and recovery process, but if your loved one has reached a terminal stage, ANH has no benefit that justifies the risk of bringing about more suffering in their final days.
- Multiple medical studies have shown that survival rates for terminally ill patients are no different if they receive ANH or not.
- Your loved one will *not* die of starvation or dehydration. They will die from their underlying condition.
- Studies have shown that IV hydration is not effective in alleviating thirst.
- ANH is administered through technical medical procedures. Like all medical procedures, there is a risk of infection.
- There are four basic ANH systems. Each has its specific risks associated with the system. These are the three most common:

---

[14] From Angela Morrow, RN

o Total Parental Nutrition (TPN): delivered through a central line, which is usually inserted at the neck or upper chest and threaded into a vein. The insert site is prone to infection. This is infection *near the heart*. (You can probably imagine how much that would suck.) Also, the central line is an imperfect device with its own set of issues, so it's not guaranteed to deliver the nutrition it's supposed to.

o Intravenous Hydration (IV): delivered through a small needle inserted into a vein and hooked up to tubing. Susceptible to infection at the insertion site or in the blood. Fluid overload can lead to significant breathing problems.

o Nastrogastric Tubes (NG): delivered through a tube inserted through the nose, down the throat, and into the stomach. If regurgitation sets in and the person is unaware and is missing the impulse to lean forward or to the side to throw up, the ANH content comes back down through the trachea and travels into the lungs. This causes an "aspiration pneumonia" – their lungs fill with vomit and they drown. (How humane is ANH sounding now?)

o Jejunostomy Tubes (J-tube): surgically inserted through the abdomen and into the jejunum (the second part of the small intestine). Provides nutrition through a bag of formula at the end of a length of tubing. Insertion procedure exposes the patient to serious risk: Surgeons punch a hole through the skin and into the stomach; this can lead to leaking of stomach contents into the abdomen, which can cause severe infection and even death. Also, just as with NG, aspiration pneumonia is a serious threat.

- Hospice workers have noticed that patients who are not tube fed seem more comfortable than those who are. Caregivers have also observed that symptoms such as nausea, vomiting, abdominal pain, incontinence, congestion, and shortness of breath—among others—decreased when artificial nutrition and hydration were discontinued, making the patient more comfortable.
- Loss of appetite is a normal part of the dying process. Nearly all terminal patients stop eating and drinking at some point. Patients and caregivers have reported that hunger is a non-issue. When it's dying, the body has no need for food; it only burdens the natural shutting-down process.

This last point is probably the most important.

RANDOM FACT: IN AUSTRALIA, SPEEDOS ARE CALLED "BUDGY SMUGGLERS," A TERM WHICH IS DERIVED FROM THE NAME OF A SMALL PARROT—THE DOMESTIC BUDGERIGAR. APPARENTLY, THE BODY-HUGGING SWIMWEAR LOOKS AS IF IT IS ATTEMPTING TO CONCEAL A PARROT WHEN VIEWED FROM THE FRONT.

This is forced feeding. The body doesn't want it. I don't know how, but the body seems to somehow know that, at this point, there is no expectation of recovery and discontinues its need for food.

Talking about this issue, despite how morbid you may think it is, is absolutely necessary. Your personal or religious convictions may lead you to believe that your loved one must receive ANH, regardless of their prognosis or level of suffering. I totally get it. Providing food and water to the suffering seems like the upright thing for you to do. But are you sure your mom or dad shares this point of view? They may see it like a lot of people do, that it's natural for the body to lose its need for food and water as it prepares for death.

Let's take a look at the animal kingdom to illustrate my point. When an animal is dying, they will find a comfortable place to curl up and sleep. You will not see the rest of the pack forcing them to eat. They all seem to see this for what it is - a natural conclusion. The dying animal takes its rest and prepares to pass peacefully.

So why don't we do the same?

We live in an age of amazing technology. Science has given us the tools to stretch out life well past the point of its natural limit, but nature will still win out in the end; it responds with weapons like organ failure and coma to reclaim its dominion over us. Our fear of death keeps us engaged in a war we cannot win. There is nothing we can do to stave off death forever. In this case, I feel it's best to do as the animals do – take your rest and prepare to pass peacefully.

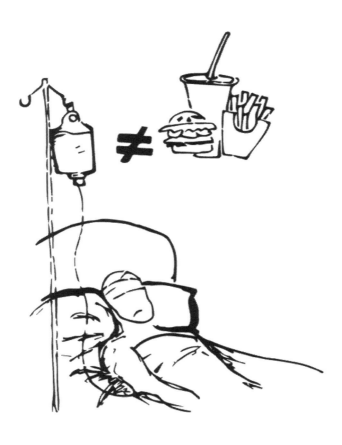

Am I asking you to forsake modern medicine and submit to nature without a fight? Absolutely not. I believe every one of us has a duty to live life as boldly as we possibly can! I only ask that you have the sense to know when it's time, and that you then focus on spending those remaining days as comfortably as possible, in dignity.

Now it's time to talk to your parent about ANH. If they decide they don't want to risk the given and possible downsides of ANH, then they should complete the form at the end of this chapter and file it with their advance directive.

RANDOM FACT: THE ANCIENT GREEKS BELIEVED THAT REDHEADS WOULD TURN INTO VAMPIRES AFTER THEY DIED.

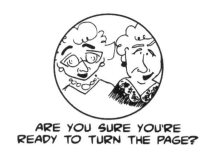

THE TALKING POINTS

Here are the points you need to be sure to bring up in your ANH discussion.

- ANH may be effective at keeping terminal patients alive for a time.
- However, studies have shown it may do little for survival rates.
- There is a serious risk of infection with all methods of ANH.
- Infection may make a patient's final days very painful and stressful.
- Loss of appetite is a natural part of the dying process.
- Hospice workers say patients who do not receive ANH are more comfortable when they pass.

My Position Regarding Artificial Nutrition and Hydration

I_____,
understand what Artificial Nutrition and Hydration (ANH) is and what it does.

I understand there are significant risks inherent in the ANH process, and I have weighed the benefits against these risks.

I have made the informed decision that I would like/ would not like (circle one) an ANH method to sustain my life in the event I am no longer able to eat or drink on my own. I do/do not (circle one) instructions as to when this may be discontinued.

I have discussed this issue with my family and the individual to whom I have assigned Power of Attorney (POA).

I will place copies of this document with my advance directive and personal will. My doctor, spouse, family, and POA all know where my paper work is.

Signed_____Date_____

(Your Signature)

Witnessed_____Date_____

(Witness's Signature)

HOME

6 CHANGING RELATIONSHIPS

Before we delve into the complexities of the family dynamic, let's take a look at a hypothetical:

Jeanie is a busy 43 year-old working mother of three teenagers. She would describe her life as hectic but good.

After her 71 year-old mother had a bad fall in her kitchen that limited her mobility, Jeanie and her husband invited her to move in with them. They felt it was their responsibility to help her out, and they took her in, despite knowing that this would be a difficult transition for all of them.

Jeanie's mom was very strict with her, but from childhood Jeanie swore she would never be that way with her own kids, and she isn't. This drives her mother crazy, so they always argue. What Jeanie really wants is for her mom to understand is that she isn't the matriarch here—her reign as mother ended decades ago. What her mom wants Jeanie to know is that she's just looking out for her grandchildren. Neither of them can figure out a way to communicate these things, so they fight.

After a year or so, Jeanie's mom's health begins to deteriorate, and she comes to rely on Jeanie for more help than she's comfortable receiving. Jeanie is starting to feel like she has another child to take care of. Both are embarrassed by how they're feeling, so they make no effort to communicate these things.

But what really has Jeanie steamed is her brother and sister's lack of contribution to their mother's welfare. Jeanie was the oldest and the loudest, so growing up they just stayed out of her way. Now she needs their help—it's their mother, too—and they're nowhere to be found. She's starting to resent them, but when she tries to communicate how she's feeling, their defensiveness just enrages her.

So, what's a busy mom and daughter to do?

RANDOM FACT: IN QUITMAN, GEORGIA, CHICKENS MAY NOT CROSS THE ROAD.

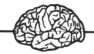

DID YOU KNOW?

According to the AARP, 64 million Americans (more than a quarter of the population) spend at least 20 hours every week taking care of sick friends, disabled family members, or an aging parent.

U.S. Department of Labor reports that approximately 30% of the American workforce are caring for an aging parent. 70% of caregivers who have jobs suffer from work-related difficulties du to their dual role as employee and caregiver.

Relationships are dynamic; over time, they grow and change, just as we do. And just like us, each one is different. Some relationships are simple, and some are . . . complicated.

What's the dynamic between you and your postman? If you're anything like me, it's probably one of limited interaction. We say hello, and he gives me my mail. It's civil and simple. Now, let's compare it to your relationship with your mother. Not quite as simple, is it? In fact, there is probably no other relationship as dynamic (and complicated) as that of parent and child.

Mosby's Medical Dictionary defines *family dynamics* as "the forces at work within a family that produce particular behaviors or symptoms." It is the way in which a family lives and interacts that defines this dynamic. And this dynamic, be it good or bad, runs so deep through us that it structures the way we interact with the world. In short, your role in this dynamic defines you as a person.

As I said earlier, relationships naturally change over time, but now with your aging parent starting to rely on you more for assistance, change just got a turbo boost.

Here's the deal: Parents begin this relationship with full control over their children. Over time, this degree of control is reduced until the children move into adulthood and have children of their own. But for most parents, there will always remain a desire to have at least some influence over their children; It's just their nature.

In Jeanie's case, her mother knows very well she is not the children's parent, but she nevertheless wants to ensure that her daughter's children are raised properly (at least by her standards). Jeanie and her mother both have maternal natures and ultimately want what's best for the kids, but this new dynamic only has room for one mother. Jeanie needs to communicate to her mother that she can't help but see this as interference. Her mother needs to recognize her daughter's authority.

So what role does her mom play in this new dynamic? She will always be Jeanie's mother, but her role is now that of Jeanie's companion. In order for this relationship to work, she must come to perceive and accept Jeanie as her *equal*—she's not her little girl anymore; Jeanie is a grown woman, and this is her home. This *woman* has chosen to open her home to a dear friend in need, *not* hand over the reins guiding her family.

However, if this new dynamic is to remain healthy, Jeanie has to give a little, too. She has to see this woman as a source of knowledge and

RANDOM FACT: WHILE IT IS A MYTH THAT STRESS CAN TURN HAIR GRAY, STRESS CAN CAUSE HAIR LOSS.

counsel. This fact will endure: Jeanie has never gone through motherhood before; she would do well to consider the advice of her trusted friend.

Sometimes, health and/or finances may force the parent to depend on their adult child for support. Jeanie's mom suffered a fall that now limits her mobility. This once proud woman has to ask her child for help. It's probably embarrassing; in fact, I'd wager that her mother considered trying to "tough it out" on her own for some time before calling her daughter. Therefore, it's very important that Jeanie perceives her mother's coming to her, despite the mortifying embarrassment, as a beautiful display of trust. A woman's dignity is at stake.

I'd like to address one more thing before we move on: You are under no obligation to help your elderly parent(s), and you should only do so if you want to. In fact, according to the National Center for Biotechnology Information, the adult child *must* identify their need to help their parent as arising from *gratitude* or *friendship* and not *debt* to avoid resenting that parent. If the adult child perceives this as debt, then, by extension, the parent is perceived as a debt-holder, and nobody likes it when the creditors come calling.

The pre-existing condition of this dynamic will definitely factor into your decision to help them or not, so if they treated you well, you'll likely want to get involved.[15] Even if they didn't treat you well, you still might want to consider it – it's an opportunity to "heal old wounds." In fact, it's your last opportunity to do so. You may become a better person for showing compassion when you received none.

This won't be an easy decision to make. There are a number of factors you need to consider – money, time, feelings, schedules, etc. Sit down with your spouse, and maybe even your children, and talk it through; it will affect all of you.

If, after careful consideration, you decide to open your home to your mom or dad, please read the next chapter very carefully, maybe even twice, to make a plan for domestic harmony. Trust me, you'll be glad you did.

There is one more relationship to consider before we move on. Remember Jeanie's frustration with her brother and sister? When she was making the decision to take her mother into her home, Jeanie neglected to do one very important thing – talk to them about it. If her brother and sister weren't involved in the decision making process, it's a little unreasonable for Jeanie to then expect them contribute to the caretaking. What she needs is a team, but teammates are only worth having when

---

[15] This may be something to bear in mind when dealing with your own children.

they're playing voluntarily, you know what I mean?

Further, Jeanie's brother and sister have always known her as the "boss." She was the oldest and a natural leader, but things have changed. Their mom needs help selling the house and wrapping up their dad's affairs. In this story, Jeanie's brother is a realtor and her sister is a lawyer. When putting together their plan, they need to forget about the old sibling dynamic. This is a new dynamic, and each sibling should contribute according to his or her strengths. Jeanie's no longer the "boss;" they're all adults, and they each have their own skill-sets.

Recognizing this, is important for the additional reason that sometimes in these situations, sibling rivalry returns to rear its ugly head once more. I honestly don't know why or how this happens, but I've seen siblings suddenly renew their fierce competition for mom's affection, despite the fact that they are now sophisticated adults. When things get heated, just do the grown-up thing: step back, take a breath, and remember you're not seven anymore, okay?

This new family dynamic is certainly complicated, but communication and consideration can make it work. I know; I went through it—twice.

RANDOM FACT: IN JUNE 2006, THE OXFORD ENGLISH DICTIONARY ADDED "GOOGLE" AS A VERB.

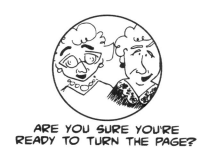

ARE YOU SURE YOU'RE
READY TO TURN THE PAGE?

THE TALKING POINTS

These are the things to bear in mind when discussing the status of your parent-child dynamic.

- Your relationship is not like it once was. You will always be their offspring, but you are no longer their child.
- You are not obligated to assist them. You must *choose* to do so.
- Even if parent-child the dynamic was negative, choosing to help your parent in their time of need is a potential way to "heal old wounds."
- The relationship with your siblings has changed, too. In order to gain their assistance in the care of your elderly parent, you must respect them as adults and recognize them as equals.

RANDOM FACT: MOTHERS WHO ARE OVER 40 AT THE TIME OF A CHILD'S BIRTH ARE 128% MORE LIKELY TO HAVE A LEFT-HANDED BABY THAN A WOMAN IN HER 20S.

7 THE LIVING SITUATION

My mother was a stubborn woman, sometimes painfully so, but I can't fault her for that. She managed to survive World War II in Germany and the Soviet occupation of Lithuania through sheer strength of will. Unremitting threats of violence and starvation surrounded her for years, but she stared them down with a steely gaze. And, yet, when the time came for her to sell our family home because she was no longer able to maintain it and herself alone, she moaned like a child.

Look, your mom or dad leaving the place that has been their (and their children's) home for so many years—simply because they can no longer keep it going on their own or they need more direct access to care—is a terrible proposition, but it's really just a house. Trust me, the grandkids would prefer to visit grandma somewhere other than the now-derelict family home that will require your well-deserved vacation time to paint, clean, and update.

Many seniors I meet maintain the romantic notion that, no matter what their needs, they will die in their own home, independent until that final hour. Sure, they might be able to pull this off, but going through such hardship unnecessarily seems sad to me. I mean, what does it really gain you? Holding on to what once was simply because it's familiar, regardless of the hardship this could heap on your family could be considered cruel.

Sometimes, you just have to let go. My mother-in-law nailed it - *A baby clenches its fists to grab all it can, but when you die, your hands are open.*

That said, I recognize that not all seniors will have to go through this. Some, in fact, *will* die in their own homes, independent until that final hour. But those situations are rare. Extraordinarily good genes, or maybe just pure luck, keeps those seniors in such good health that they won't need to make this kind of adjustment to their living situation. However, chances are your mom or dad won't be one of them.

It's very important that you talk about this subject with your parent *now*, while they're more inclined to be objective. Waiting to talk about it until the need for alternative living arrangements arises is a really bad idea, as that will most likely be a far more emotional time in both your lives.

After you've brought up the topic with your elderly parent, it's a good idea to take a look at your options. Not everyone will need the same amount of care and each option has its pros and cons, so there really is no one-size-fits-all solution here.

This chapter will cover the three most common alternative living options: in your home, in an Assisted Living Facility, and in a Shared Home. You and your parent should consider each one and find the one that's right for both of you.

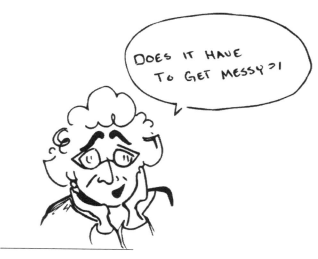

IN YOUR HOME

This is perhaps both the simplest and the most complicated option we'll discuss. As discussed in the previous chapter, *Changing Relationships*, when an elderly parent comes to rely on their adult child to a greater extent due to need, the parent-child relationship dynamic is greatly affected. This paradigm shift opens the door to confusion and resentment, and, really, the only shot you have at avoiding these is to have a candid conversation about what's going to happen, and how it will make you feel.

Your relationship with your parent is not what it once was – you're a grownup with your own family. Therefore, it's your house and these are your rules. I realize this puts you in uncharted territory, so let's make a map.

First, your new resident(s) must respect your authority, especially when it comes to raising your children. I can't tell you how many times I butted heads with my mother on this one. A mother's nature really never changes, so even in her eighties she was still determined to be the matriarch. However, my children had *their* mother, and it wasn't her. This must be a steadfast rule: *only one mother at a time*. Why? Think about it from your kids' perspective – Mom was Mom and Grandma was Grandma. Now, Grandma's living with them and sharing Mom's duties. It's confusing and, I'll bet, more than just a little frustrating.

Second, *everyone* will contribute something to the household. I'm not saying you should sentence your mother to hard labor, but I will say that when my mom was busy in the garden, she seemed content to lay off scrutinizing my parenting for a couple hours. By letting your parent do even little chores around the house, two things are accomplished: 1) chores and 2) they begin to feel like a contributing party, and not just a long-term guest. When your parent feels like a *member* of your household, they'll never feel like a *burden* on the household; that's important because you don't want to have a mopey senior wandering your hallway—you want a motivated member of the team."/>

Along similar lines, you want them to commit to maintaining independence by remaining active. Is there a hobby they've always wanted to take up but never had the time? Now is the perfect time to learn

---

"/>RANDOM FACT: OF THE 10,000 SPECIES OF MUSHROOMS, ONLY 250 ARE EDIBLE.

line dancing, or maybe help with some carpentry! Chances are good that there is a senior center near you. Contact them to see what services they offer. Also, check out the local community college for continuing education classes. (The one near me even offers scuba diving!)

The final thing[16] to discuss before jumping into the logistics of sharing your home is the emotional aspect. Acknowledge to your mom or dad and yourself that you don't have a clue what you're doing. There is no formal training that can prepare you for dealing with this situation, so you're going into this thing blind. Admit you're scared. Then, acknowledge that the only way everyone will get through this is to do it together and to live by a plan. Yes, things will change as this "inter-generational cohabitation experiment" progresses, so you should be prepared to make small changes on the fly, but a solid plan can save you from a 3 a.m. chocolate ice cream breakdown. Trust me. Read the rest of the chapter. Figure out the logistics. Delegate duties. Write it down. Et voilà! A plan!

---

[16] Actually, a *second* final thing: be sure to have your kids spend some time with the grandparent. They will learn valuable life lessons and important bits of family history that they might not get from their parents.

Now, on to the adventures that await!

Housing

Moving mom or dad into your home won't be as simple as it was moving yourself. There are a number of considerations that need to be addressed. First, what are their needs? Will they need a wheelchair ramp? Do you anticipate needing one? What do they need in a bathroom? (Do they take baths or showers? Will they need rails near the toilet?)

Then, you've got to think about "senior-proofing" the house; yes, it's a lot like baby-proofing. Pay attention to sharp edges on corners and loose cords they could trip on.

Next, what privacy accommodations will they require? Can they share a bathroom? Will you need to convert a living room into a bedroom to accommodate medical equipment? If so, can you have doors installed to close off the area when they need some space? Do they need their own entrance/exit?

Lastly, what are you going to do with all of

RANDOM FACT: IN MICHIGAN, A WOMAN'S HAIR BELONGS TO HER HUSBAND.

their belongings? If your husband is anything like mine, your garage is probably already overflowing with stuff. Where would you find the space to put your mom's treasured knickknacks or sentimental linens? Should you rent a storage unit? Who's responsible for that? Is she open to reducing the inventory a bit? It's a lifetime of accumulation, but most of it is just *stuff*. Sometimes getting ready for a garage sale can help a senior reorganize their lives – when you can no longer have it all, you have to consider what's really important to you.

Something to bear in mind here – it's a bit traumatic to let go of your prized possessions at a garage sale, so the kind thing to do might be to arrange for your parent to be somewhere else and not tell them what things sold for upon their return. It is shocking how little those personal treasures are worth on the open market.

Finances[17]

It's really important that both of you come to understand the state of your parent's finances, as money is probably the number one thing you two will argue about. (Nothing really ever changes.)

---

[17] This section is important to discuss regardless of which housing option works best for your situation.

What are the sources of income? Do they have a pension? What about social security? A 401K? On a related issue, what contributions from other family members can you count on? Would your siblings pledge a certain amount of money every month to cover mom's care?

After you've grasped the income part, it's time to talk expenditures.

Money is inextricably linked to a sense of independence, so it's really important that you let your mom or dad pay for as much of their care as they are reasonably able. Remember that mopey senior wandering your hallway I mentioned earlier? I wasn't trying to be funny. Although adult children think they're honoring mom by taking care of everything for her, they may not be. She needs to maintain a sense of independence, even while transitioning to a state of greater dependence, in order to "keep her chin up." The easiest (and cheapest) way to do this is to create a budget for mom, with *her* sources of income providing much of the funding.

Fire up Excel and make a spreadsheet. Be sure to account for every expense that you can foresee, and leave a little cushion for the unforeseeable. List all mom's income sources. With the numbers there in front of you at the table, you two will be able to make informed decisions.

(One quick note before moving on: Otherwise trusting people sometimes become quite paranoid when it comes to their money. It's important that you not only keep this accounting up to date but also make it readily available to those who might need to see it. Siblings, in particular, might need to be convinced you're not spending mom's money on yourself. I've seen it happen.)

Healthcare Plan

Seniors spend a lot of time with healthcare professionals; it's a simple fact. Given this, why, *oh why*, do doctor visits always seem to come as a complete surprise to the adult children? It's called a "calendar," and it's not very expensive. Hell, I've even got one on my phone. Get one and *use it*. Don't let these things catch you by surprise. Create a schedule with your parent and task them with keeping it updated and you informed. Also, make them aware that *they* are responsible for

---

RANDOM FACT: GOLD IS SO RARE THAT THE WORLD POURS MORE STEEL IN AN HOUR THAN IT HAS POURED GOLD SINCE THE BEGINNING OF RECORDED HISTORY.

coordinating transportation if they don't drive. A heads-up call from them an hour before the appointment would be appreciated too!

One more thing about this before moving on – make sure they don't skip appointments. You might think, "oh, it's just a doctor's appointment," but it's a little more complicated than that. The doctor has created and wants to keep a healthcare *plan* for your parent. Treatments for seniors are generally not one-time things—each appointment *matters*. When the goal is to maintain a complicated care approach, letting mom miss an appointment just because she she'd rather not go abrogates the hard work of her healthcare *partner*. (FYI: When that healthcare partner is *me*, I'm not as nice about it as people expect.)

Documents[18]

Seniors come with lots of paperwork – just another fact of life. If a senior is moving into your home, one of the first things you will need to do is to make a trip to your local office supply store. You're going to need one of those accordion

---

[18] If you're looking at an Assisted Living Facility instead of your home, ask the Director of Nursing if s/he will maintain this folder for you.

folders. Be sure it's the kind with tabs.

Once you have the folder, you're going to want to make the following tabs:

- Medical Records
- Advance Directive/Living Will
- DNR (if applicable)
- Will
- Receipts

Then, file the paperwork behind the corresponding tab.

When that's finished, you should take a piece of printer paper, fold it in half and tape it to the front of the folder. On this half-sheet you should have your parent write following:

- My doctor is: _____

  Phone: _____

- Power of Attorney is: _____

  Phone: _____

- My Executor is: _____

  Phone: _____

- I have (or don't have) DNR.

- My current prescriptions are:

  _____

_____

_____

- My allergies are:

_____

_____

**If you have a scanner available, it is always
smart to have a backup on file as well as other
important documents, such as passports, credit
cards, marriage certificates, etc.**

Transportation

If your parent has given up their keys, then
your family will have to step up to make sure they
can still get to where they need to go. I know you
didn't go to college to become a chauffeur, but if
everyone with a driver's license agrees to do a part
of the driving, your parent can avoid being stuck at
home with little inconvenience for each of you.
Create a weekly schedule of where they need to be
and when, and then coordinate calendars with the
other drivers.

Conferences

As I advised before, it's very important that you

discuss the above-mentioned concerns before they arise, but it's equally important that you maintain a dialogue after your mom or dad moves into your home. Issues will arise, and things will change. You will all need to keep on top of all of this if you want to maintain a peaceful home.

Set up regular family conferences to keep everyone up-to-speed. I always suggest Sunday dinners, as this seems to be a convenient and relaxed time for most of us. Make sure everyone is present and ready to talk. Be sure to address upcoming events and appointments. Also, be prepared to talk about how you're feeling – pent-up emotions can lead to resentment. Be civil, but be honest. This is all about getting along for the long haul.

Relief

This is a really important topic, and it's one that often goes ignored, despite being of vital importance. You're not a martyr; you will need a break from time-to-time. Make sure you get one. Want to stay married? Be sure to have "date night." In fact, demand it. Coordinate with your siblings to, at the very least, get rotating Saturday nights.

Also, stay on those siblings to remain engaged

in your parent's life by taking them on occasional outings or maybe weekends at their place. It's important that they don't come to associate mom or dad as being just another part of your household—seniors don't become the sole property of the offspring who takes them in. In the words of the celebrated purple philosopher, Barney, *caring is sharing.*

ASSISTED LIVING FACILITY

Let's quickly revisit an important point: It is unrealistic for your senior parent to think they can live on their own without assistance forever. If they don't want to move into your home at some point, you two will have to come up with a plan for where they will go when they've reached the point that they can no longer meet their own daily needs. A good alternative is something called an Assisted Living Facility.

"Assisted living" is a type of care designed for people who are able to live and function on their own, but who need some assistance with activities of daily living (ADL). Assisted living care typically

---

RANDOM FACT: MORE THAN 80 SPELLING VARIATIONS ARE RECORDED FOR SHAKESPEARE'S NAME, FROM "SHAPPERE" TO "SHAXBERD."

involves meal preparation, some housekeeping and laundry services, and may also include personal assistance with bathing, dressing, ambulating, and medication. For seniors suffering from dementia, some senior assisted living communities have memory care units specially equipped with safety features. Oftentimes, these assisted living homes also offer memory care programs customized to maintain or improve cognitive function for assisted living residents.[19]

This may be a happy medium for you if your mom or dad wishes to maintain as much independence as possible, while remaining in a stimulating environment. They would live in a community of seniors—a very beneficial setting, as it's always great to be around people who know exactly what you're going through when you're making a tough transition. Assisted living facilities also offer a lot of social activities specifically for seniors as well—many have an activities coordinator whose primary job is to plan fun things for the residents to do together.

But I'll be honest with you here – while most of the seniors I've talked to have really enjoyed

---

[19] From assistedlivingsource.com, a great place to begin your search.

their assisted living experiences, there are a few whose time there they would describe as less than great. That's why it's important to do your homework when looking for an assisted living residence. I'll go into more detail on how to do that in the later chapter entitled *The Pledge to Age Bravely*, but I'll give you a condensed version here.

First, visit *at least* three different facilities and get to know the staff a little at each one. While you're there, be sure to ask all of your questions. *Do not be embarrassed!* These facilities want your business, so you're in charge of your visit and can inquire about anything you want. Got it?

Here's a list of questions you should definitely ask:

- What types of services are offered here?
  - Meal preparation, Housekeeping, Laundry, and Personal Assistance?
  - Aides and Nurses/Nurse Practitioner?
  - Emergency response?
- Is the medical staff certified?
- How regularly are you inspected? What accreditations do you have?
- What is your "philosophy of care"?
- How old is the facility? Is it regularly maintained?

- How's the food? Will you accommodate dietary restrictions?
- Are religious services offered?
- If applicable – what are your dementia and/or immobility provisions?[20]
- What is your visitation policy? Hours?[21]
- Can I come by after-hours to see what it's like at night?

With that out of the way, it's time to talk about your individual findings. Weigh the pros and cons of each facility you visited. Be sure to discuss your "gut feelings" about the place – some things are immeasurable. Also, consider the logistics of the move to one of these places – How would they move in? Will their room have enough space to fit the things they can't live without? What will they do with the rest?

Then, it's time for you, the adult child, to talk about the guilt you're feeling. Don't lie; I know you're feeling some. Nobody wants to be the bad

---

[20] If these facilities won't handle advanced dementia, you may have to consider custodial care, aka "Nursing Homes,", which, with their in-house medical staff, are better equipped to provide this kind of care.

[21] Consider the compatibility of this answer with whether this is a reasonable distance for family members to travel and if these hours are convenient.

guy who put mom in a "home." It's completely normal to feel this way, but you know what? You're a grown up and, together with your mom or dad, you made a grownup decision. You are *not* "warehousing" them. You found a way to get them the care they can no longer provide for themselves, despite the enormous emotional impact it has had on you. If there has ever been a greater display of love for a parent, I haven't seen it.

Finally, you need to stay engaged. I know you're super busy, but just because your mom isn't in your home doesn't mean she shouldn't be a part of your daily life. Get her a cell phone. If she doesn't already know how, teach her how to send text messages and pictures from her new life. Visit whenever you can, and, for the love of God, bring her some flowers!

IN A SHARED HOME

If your parent simply *will not* leave their home, don't fret – you've still got one more option: shared homes.

A common justification used by seniors who can no longer meet their own needs, but are nevertheless unwilling to leave their homes, is that "this house is paid for!" While that may be true, what they're failing to account for (excuse the pun) is the day-to-day expenses inherent in homeownership. This can be expensive—not just in terms of cash but also labor, and the expense is often too much for one senior to handle.

So what can they do? They can share the expense of keeping up their home by taking in other seniors and pooling their resources. We called this "shared living," which essentially creates a senior community in an environment that's most comfortable to them. It also provides "safety in numbers" – a "seniors taking care of seniors" situation.

When you propose this idea (or, for that matter, the assisted living option), you may hear a couple of different snarky responses. My favorite one is this: "I don't want to live with a bunch of old fogies!" To which I would likely respond, "Would you rather be hanging out at the mall with my kids? Besides, *somebody* needs to keep an eye on those old fogies."

RANDOM FACT: MARS' RED COLOR IS DUE TO IRON OXIDE, ALSO KNOWN AS RUST, AND IT'S SOIL HAS THE CONSISTENCY OF TALCUM POWDER. LITERALLY, THE METALLIC ROCKS ON MARS ARE RUSTING.

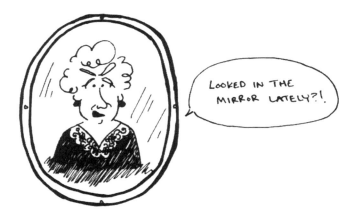

This is the indisputable truth: The decline of their health will likely force them to make some sort of compromise—that's not up for debate—but they do have options.

Your task as the concerned loved one is to find a way to get them to be reasonable about this. It's never easy, but I have faith in you.

RANDOM FACT: TEN-YEAR-OLD JACK SINGER OF WARWICK, NEW YORK, WORE 215 PAIRS OF UNDERWEAR SIMULTANEOUSLY ON JUNE 13, 2010. HE BROKE THE PREVIOUS RECORD OF 200 PAIRS.

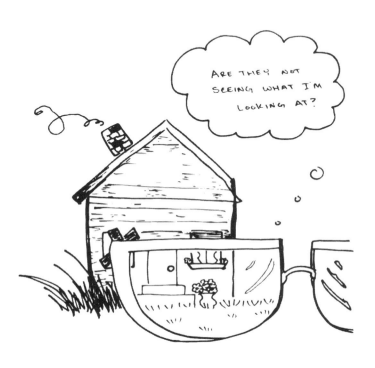

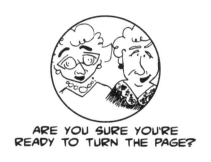

THE TALKING POINTS

There will likely come a day when your elderly parent won't be able to safely live on their own. When that day comes, the family needs to have a plan. Luckily, there are a number of options to consider.

- Moving in with the adult children – things to consider:
  - New Dynamic – respect each other as adults, and love each other as family.
  - Parenting – the children have a mother and father already; these roles must be respected.
  - Accommodations – figure out what will work for all of you (and what to do with all of the personal belongings).
  - "Senior Proofing" – modifications to the home may need to be made in order to accommodate certain needs.
  - Communication – be ready to share openly and honestly at regular family meetings to keep peace in the home. All

of you are going through a significant change. Talk about it to keep your sanity!
  - ○ Participation – everyone contributes in the day-to-day operations of the home. Define everyone's role in this.
  - ○ Care partners – involve your siblings in the parent's care. Be sure to get some time for "date night" to maintain sanity.
- Assisted Living Facility – things to consider
  - ○ Adjustment – you would be living in a senior *community*, thus, you will not be the matriarch or patriarch. You will be part of a system.
  - ○ Options – like buying a car, you have choices to fit your tastes and budget. There are a few lemons out there, though, so be sure to check them out thoroughly.
- A Shared Home – things to consider
  - ○ This might be a happy medium. You maintain more independence through pooled resources. However, be realistic about what you can accomplish with the physical and financial limitations the members of the household might have.

Just like asking a senior to stop driving when they can no longer drive safely, asking a senior to consider changing their living situation will be met with fierce resistance. Things to discuss:

- Ignoring your physical limitations that may prevent you from living on your own is, in fact, ignoring reality.
- Are you *really* capable of doing the things you need to do to keep up the house?
    - Mowing the lawn? Walking the dog? Cleaning the kitty litter? Vacuuming?
- If you're all alone, what's your plan in case of a serious fall? How will you get help if you can't reach the phone?

8 SENIORS BEHIND THE WHEEL

When my son was about twelve years old, he and his sisters went to stay with my mother for the summer. One day I called just to see how they were doing. Mom and I chatted casually for a little bit before I asked to speak with the kids. When it was Jon's turn to talk, he was so excited that he could barely breathe.[22] "Mom!" he exclaimed, "Grandma ran her car through the garage door today!" While I could see how this would be thrilling for a child, *I* didn't quite see it that way. "Put grandma back on the phone," I said.

In fairness to my mother, I could see how, with a car full of kids as rambunctious as mine, one could fail to remember that backing the car out of the driveway requires putting the car in *Reverse* and not *Drive*. I could have, as her insurance company mercifully did, written the whole thing off as a random accident. But I saw the problem coming up on the horizon. When she graduated from garage doors to gas pumps, I knew it was time to have a

---

[22] It is important to note that Jon still gets this excited on the phone, but it was only cute when he was twelve.

little chat.

The day had come for my mom to give up her driver's license, and she knew it, but she'd be damned if she was going to hand it over without a fight.

Ever since most of us were sixteen years old, that license has been something of our own personal Declaration of Independence.[23] The minute you got this little card from your local DMV, you were liberated from the shackles of parental tyranny (or so it seemed for about a day). You were free to roam! Road trips! Drive-ins! Tailgating! So many of our greatest memories are directly linked to that laminated liberator. And now, you're going to have to ask your parent to hand it over. Of course they're going to resist, but as we'll see, the facts speak for themselves–seniors and cars can be a dangerous combination.

In this chapter, I'll be preparing you for an epic battle. Both sides are going to fight like hell to get their way on this one, but common sense *has* to prevail. If you objectively assess your senior driver's ability to stay on the road, and you arrive at the conclusion that they're no longer safe to drive, they've *got* to hand the keys over – if not for their own safety, then for that of everyone else on the road.

---

[23] Cue the National Anthem.

Seniors have surpassed teenagers as the fastest growing segment of the driving population. In 2006, the National Highway Traffic Safety Administration reported that more than 30 million people over the age of 65 were licensed drivers in the U.S. This group now represents 15 percent of all licensed drivers in this country.

According to David Rosenfield, an editor at the *Elder Law Journal*, drivers 75 and older have a 37 percent higher crash rate than teenage drivers. When another vehicle is involved in a crash, approximately 72 percent of the time that second party will be a senior. Seniors account for 14 percent of all individuals killed in automobile accidents. In Florida alone, a national transportation research group found that 271 of the 503 drivers who died in accidents in 2010 were senior drivers.

Now, let's take a look at *why* seniors and risk sometimes travel our roads together.

As we've discussed in previous chapters, seniors are going through a phase of mental and physical change. Some of these changes lead to factors that expose them to danger when behind the wheel.[24] These factors include:

- Slower reaction time
- Depth perception/general vision changes

---

[24] From seniors.lovetoknow.com, a great site with all sorts of helpful advice.

- Hearing problems
- Decreased ability to focus mentally
- Feelings of nervousness and anxiety
- Side effects of medication

These factors, while bothersome at home, can be deadly on the road. Unfortunately, the task of recognizing when one or more of these factors have affected a senior driver to the extent that they're no longer safe behind the wheel, falls almost completely on the shoulders of the drivers and their families.

There are no federal laws governing senior driving, and the states cannot seem to agree on a method for assessing senior driver risk. In many states, no special consideration is paid to senior drivers. In fact, in the majority of states, if the driver has a valid license and insurance, the state has no issue with them driving.[25] Only *two* states[26] require senior drivers to pass a road test to renew their licenses. I hate to sound melodramatic, but in a way, those other 48 states have blood on their hands.

Katie Bolka was a high school junior in Dallas on her way to take an algebra test when Elizabeth

---

[25] In fairness, the State of Florida requires the driver to be breathing for the duration of the trip.

[26] Illinois and New Hampshire require seniors to complete a driving test with an in-car evaluator to renew their licenses.

Grimes, 90, mistook the accelerator for the brake. Grimes barreled through a red light and struck Katie's car. Katie fought for five days but eventually succumbed to her injuries.

Here's the kick in the teeth: Grimes had been in accident just prior to this one and even continued to drive after Katie's death.

This outrage has compelled Rick Bolka, Katie's father, to act. He has been pushing the Texas senate to pass a bill that would toughen the state's laws on risky senior drivers. "[T]he first level of defense is the driver," he said.[27] "The second level of defense is the (driver's) family. The third level of defense is the (driver's) physician. We would like to see the state become the first level of defense. The government has a responsibility to protect its citizens."

To perfectly illustrate Bolka's point, Texas Sen. John Corona, R-Dallas, said during a hearing that his mother "is blind, and they just renewed her license by mail."

But it looks like Texas is going to do something about it. Bolka's bill will likely be signed into law by Governor Rick Perry, and it will require drivers 79 and older to appear in person for renewals, as well as subject them to mandatory vision tests and

---

[27] From USAToday.com

behind-the-wheel exams if officials have any question about their driving abilities. Drivers 85 and older would be required to renew every two years. (Hallelujah! Only 47 more states to go!)

"The [insurance] industry views [senior drivers] as pretty much a self-policing group. Many elderly drivers do not drive at night. Many will make three right-hand turns instead of one left-hand turn," says Carolyn Gorman, vice president of the Insurance Information Institute.[28] I hear this a lot, and I agree with her for the most part – a lot of elderly drivers pay careful attention, not only to the road but also to their own limitations. However, stubborn seniors like my mother use this justification well past the point where it stops being true. People like her, well, you may have to pry the keys from their hands, because they know damn well they've gone beyond the point where just a little extra caution will keep them safe. They know they don't belong behind the wheel anymore, but they'll continue to do or say anything to keep those keys on that key ring.

So what do we? I've given you the facts, and now I'll go over the right way and wrong way to bring it up. If you make it through all of that, I'll reward you with a couple of possible solutions for this dilemma.

---

[28] From USAToday.com

Confrontation Approach vs. Open-Ended Questions and Reflective Listening[29]

I was raised in South Boston, which, for those of you not familiar with the social mores particular to "Southie," tends to be more confrontational than much of the country. We speak our minds and tend to give little concern to how our words are received. I'm not excusing this, but it's how we were raised. In my line of work, it's called "bad bedside manner." I don't use the confrontational approach in dealing with seniors, and you shouldn't either. It often leads to conflict with very distant resolution because many seniors are capable of being quite a bit more stubborn than you (I don't know where they find the energy for such vehement defenses, but they surely do). Here's an example of how the confrontational approach can blow up in your face:

You: *You just ran that red light! Didn't you see it?*

Mom: *No, I must have missed it. Oops!*

You: *What if someone had been in that crosswalk? They'd be dead right now.*

Mom: *Nothing happened. Let it go!*

You: *What about the time you parked the car in*

---

[29] For more on this, check out Elizabeth Dugan's great book, *The Driving Dilemma.*

*the garage without opening the garage door?
You're not safe to drive anymore, Ma. You're
scaring me!*

Mom: *Do you want to walk home?!*

Look, no one would question you intentions
here. You were as afraid for your mother as you
were for that guy who wasn't in the crosswalk.
Congratulations, you're a good person. But you just
ensured you won't be able to have a civilized
conversation about her driving ever again. A topic
as sensitive as this one requires a bit of finesse.

A better strategy is to ask open-ended questions
and follow with reflective listening. The chances
are good that your mother has noticed her new
driving limitations. She's probably as concerned as
you are and might already be adjusting her driving
practice to accommodate these things. But how will
you know how she's feeling unless you get her
talking? Try this:

> You: *Mom, you seemed a bit nervous when
> we came to that intersection. How are you
> feeling about your driving?*

See what that does? You've expressed the same

RANDOM FACT: TO MAKE A CARPET BRIGHTER, SPRINKLE SALT
ONTO THE CARPET AND LET IT STAND FOR AN HOUR BEFORE
VACUUMING IT UP. SALT IS ALSO EFFECTIVE IN REMOVING MUDDY
FOOTPRINTS.

concern as you did with the confrontational approach, but you've done it in such a way that doesn't immediately place her on the defensive. If you ask her like a concerned friend, she will be inclined to answer you as such. Instead of responding with "do you want to walk home?!", you may just get unrestrained honesty:

> Mom: *You know, I'm doing okay in the daytime, but driving at night makes me really nervous. I have trouble focusing when it's dark.*

You can then respond with reflective listening to let her know that you are truly hearing what she's saying and want to help her.

> You: *Trouble focusing? Have you had your vision checked recently? It may be something as simple as adjusting your prescription.*

Now you've just identified yourself as an ally in her healthcare. The case may very well be that she will soon need to hand over the keys, but by starting a dialogue about her driving before it comes to that point, you're setting the groundwork to make that later conversation easier.

Which leads me to the solution I mentioned earlier: If you want to avoid having a cage match on your hands when you feel it's time for mom to hand over the keys, start talking about it early. Express your concerns;[30] discuss the facts. Then, bring up the Family Driving Agreement.

The Family Driving Agreement is essentially a contract designed to reinforce your family's senior safe driving plan. It acknowledges that there will come a day when the senior driver is no longer able to drive safely. It documents that a trusted friend or family member has been designated to make that determination when the time comes, and it holds that the senior driver should abide by that determination. With a Family Driving Agreement in place, the "hand over the keys" conversation will still be a rough one to have, but at least the chances are better you'll get out of it without requiring a trip to the E.R. (Who knew little old ladies had such a propensity for violence?).

---

[30] If both of you feel that the senior is still capable of being safe behind the wheel, I would still strongly suggest they take the AARP's "Driving Course for People Over 50." It provides a lot of helpful information on such topics as:
- How to make adjustments due to hearing, vision, and slower reactions
- Proper distance to maintain behind cars
- Lane changing and turn safety

Family Driving Agreement[31]

Dear family,

As I continue through the aging process, I realize there may come a day when the advantages of my continuing to drive are outweighed by the safety risk I pose, not only to myself, but also to other motorists.

I want to continue driving for as long as is safely possible, but when my driving is no longer safe, I will trust:

_____

(name of trusted friend or relative)

when he/she tells me that I need to discontinue driving, or to continue driving with certain restrictions.

I will maintain my integrity by listening to and accepting this individual's driving-related recommendations, thereby ensuring not only my safety, but also the safety of the motoring public.

Signed _____ Date _____

(As Senior Driver)

Signed _____ Date _____

(As Person Named Above Witness)

---

[31] Adapted from www.keepingussafe.org, a great site to learn about senior driving safety that is run by Matt Gurwell, a retired 24-year veteran of the Ohio State Highway Patrol.

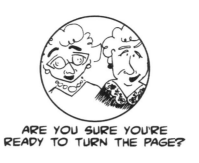

ARE YOU SURE YOU'RE
READY TO TURN THE PAGE?

THE TALKING POINTS

Before you go in there, just remember this: they won't be giving up that license without a fight. Be prepared! Review these talking points and write in your own notes in the margins.

Don't say you weren't warned.

- There will come a time for all of us when we are no longer safe to drive.
- Our need for the feeling of independence those keys provide should never be more important than your safety and the safety of those with whom we share the road.
- Signing the Family Driving Agreement would show your family that you are informed and realistic about your aging.
- The Confrontation Approach to addressing this issue is not appropriate for these discussions. Let's take turns speaking frankly and listening respectfully.

9 THE WILL THE EXECUTOR

Preface: Let me begin this section by making one thing very clear – I am not an attorney. When you sit down to write up your will and assign an executor, you would be well advised to seek the assistance of a lawyer, preferably one specializing in estate planning. At a basic level, these things are easy to understand, but there's a world of distance between understanding and effective execution. Moving on . . . .

So, what is a will? Put simply, it's a legally binding document in which you direct to whom your money and possessions go after you've passed on.

Creating a will is important for a number of reasons. The most important reason is this: *You* get

---

RANDOM FACT: WHEN HORACE AND DAEIDA WILCOX FOUNDED HOLLYWOOD IN 1887, THEY HOPED IT WOULD BECOME A RELIGIOUS COMMUNITY. PROHIBITIONISTS, THEY BANNED LIQUOR FROM THE TOWN AND OFFERED FREE LAND TO ANYONE WILLING TO BUILD A CHURCH.

to decide who gets what and when. If you die without a will, your estate is said to be "intestate," which is a really bad thing. This means the state in which you resided is responsible for tracking down your heirs and divvying up your stuff among them in a manner the *court* thinks is fair. The rules that govern the determination of these issues are called the *laws of intestate succession*, and they vary state-by-state.

For the purposes of an example of the process by which the court applies the laws of intestate succession, we'll take a look at California's series of questions the courts ask before making a ruling.[32]

1. The first question is whether the decedent (the person who died) was married.
   a. If the decedent was not married, the estate is distributed as follows:

      i. To the decedent's children, who take in equal shares if they are in the same generation.
      ii. If there are no children or other issue (issue is the legal term for children, grandchildren, great-grandchildren, etc.) living, the estate goes to the decedent's parents.

---

[32] These questions were generously provided by Stephen C. Gruber, a probate attorney in Los Altos, California.

iii. If there are no parents living, the estate is distributed to the "issue of the parents." If the decedent had brothers or sisters, they will inherit the estate. If there are deceased brothers and sisters, and they had issues, the issues will inherit the share of the estate that the deceased brother or sister would have inherited.

iv. If there are no brothers or sisters, the decedent's grandparents will inherit the estate.

v. If there are no living grandparents, then the "issue of the grandparents" will inherit the estate. This could include the decedent's aunts and uncles, or if there aren't any aunts and uncles, the decedent's cousins. Generally, the oldest generation that has surviving issue will inherit, but if there are deceased issue in that generation, their issue will inherit their share.

vi. If there are no cousins, Probate Code section 6402 provides that the estate will be distributed to "next of kin in equal degree," generally meaning more distant cousins.

b. If the decedent was married, the first question is whether the decedent owned community property, separate property, or a combination of the two.

Community property is generally defined as the assets acquired during marriage from earnings or salary. Separate property is generally defined as assets brought into the marriage when the decedent got married, inheritances to the decedent, or gifts to the decedent. However, California case law provides many exceptions to these definitions, and assets can change from community to separate property, or from separate to community, by combining assets, by improving separate property with community property, or by written agreement of the spouses, for example.

    i.   The decedent's community property goes to the surviving spouse, who may have to file a spousal property petition to establish ownership.

    ii.   The decedent's separate property is distributed as follows:

        1.   The surviving spouse receives all of the separate

RANDOM FACT: ORIGINALLY, THE TERM "MOVIES" DID NOT MEAN FILMS, BUT THE PEOPLE WHO MADE THEM. IT WAS GENERALLY USED WITH DISDAIN BY EARLY HOLLYWOOD LOCALS WHO DISLIKED THE "INVADING" EASTERNERS.

property if the decedent is not survived by issue, parents, brothers, sisters, or children of a deceased brother or sister.

2.   The surviving spouse receives one-half of the separate property if the decedent had only one child, or issue of a deceased child.

3.   The surviving spouse receives one-half of the separate property if the decedent left no issue, but left parent(s) or their issue.

4.   The surviving spouse receives <u>only one-third</u> of the separate property if the decedent left more than one child.

5.   The surviving spouse receives <u>only one-third</u> of the separate property if the decedent left one child and the issue of one or more deceased children.

6.   The surviving spouse receives <u>only one-third</u> of the separate property if the decedent left the issue of two or more deceased children.

* * * * *

Gee. Wasn't that fun? (If you answered "yes," then you're probably a probate attorney.) So, why did I include all that legal mumbo-jumbo? It's here to stress the fact that you really need to take care of these arrangements before the state has to do it for you. Think of it as the humane thing to do—going through this legal process is really unpleasant. I'm serious; it's a pretty cruel thing to do to your loved ones. Dealing with depositions and hearings and lawyers and tears—is that really what you want your kids to be doing when they should be trying to move on with their lives after mourning your loss?

One more thing about avoiding this disaster before moving on: The court doesn't give a damn about your family—well, not personally, anyway. There are laws that govern intestate succession in your state, and the court will follow those laws—regardless of whether David was an absolute angel when you were going through chemotherapy, or if Jillian was an unhinged nightmare after the divorce. They're both going to get an equal share simply because they're related to you. I know they're both your kids and you should love them all equally, but let's face it—one of your kids may be a jerk. The court has no interest in your family dynamic, but maybe you do.

So, now that I've scared you into creating your

will, let's look at an example. I've provided a copy of the Statutory Will template provided by the California State Bar. (Your state's requirements may be a little different, so check with them.) While this example is somewhat limited in its scope, it's a good model for you to use when thinking about your will.

LAST WILL AND TESTAMENT OF

_____

*I, _____, now residing in
the County of _____, State of
California, and being of sound mind and memory
and not acting under fraud, menace, duress or the
undue influence of any person whomsoever, do
hereby make, publish and declare this to be my Last
Will and Testament, and hereby expressly revoke
any and all former wills and codicils to wills
heretofore made by me.*

FIRST: *I declare that I am married to
_____, and all references in
this will to my wife are to her. I further declare that
any references in this will to my children shall
include any child of mine born from this day
forward, or legally adopted. At the present time I
have _____ children, _____,
_____, and
_____.*

SECOND: *I direct my executor, hereinafter named,
to pay all my just debts, expenses of administration,
and my last illness and funeral costs as soon after
my death as is convenient.*

THIRD: *I nominate* _____
as executor, to serve without bond. If
_____ *shall for any reason fail*
to qualify or cease to act as executor, I nominate
_____ *as executor, also to*
serve without bond. I direct that my executor take
all actions legally permissible to have the probate
of my estate done as simply as possible, including
filing a petition in the appropriate court for the
independent administration of my estate under the
California Independent Administration of Estates
Act.

Initials_____

Prior to distribution, the said personal
representative shall have in addition to those
powers conferred by law, those powers reasonably
required, including the power to sell at either public
or private sale, to mortgage, pledge, lease,
exchange or otherwise dispose of the whole, or any
part, of the real or personal property of my estate,
with or without first securing an order of Court, but
subject to any confirmation by the Court that may
be required by law. My Executor shall pay from the
residue of my estate all inheritance, estate and other
death taxes (excluding any additional tax that may
be assessed under Internal Revenue Code Section
2032(a), including interest and penalties, that may,
because of my death, be attributable to any assets

properly inventoried in my probate estate. The taxes shall be charged against my estate as though they were ordinary expenses of administration without adjustment among the beneficiaries of my Will.

FOURTH: *I hereby give, or devise and bequeath all of my property and estate, both real and personal, and wheresoever or howsoever situated, or to which I may be entitled at the time of my death, as follows:*

To my wife, _____ if my wife does not survive me by 120 hours then I give all my property to my children, to be divided into equal shares. If any of my children do not survive me by 120 hours their share shall be divided equally among my surviving children.. If none of my children do not survive me by 120 hours then I give all my property to _____. If _____ does not survive me by 120 hours then I give all my property to _____. If _____ does not survive me by 120 hours then I give all my property to _____
_____.

Initials_____

FIFTH: *If my wife and I should die simultaneously,*

or under such circumstances as to render it difficult or impossible to determine by clear and convincing evidence who predeceased the other, I shall be conclusively presumed to have survived my wife for purposes of this will.

SIXTH: *Except as otherwise provided in this Will, I have intentionally and with full knowledge omitted to provide for heirs. If any beneficiary under this Will in any manner, directly or indirectly, contests this Will or any of its provisions, any share of interest in my estate given to that contesting beneficiary under this Will is revoked and shall be disposed of in the same manner provided herein as if that contesting beneficiary had predeceased me without issue.*

IN WITNESS WHEREOF, I subscribe my name to this will this _____ day of _____, 201__ at

_____,

and do hereby declare that I sign and execute this instrument as my last will and that I sign it willingly, that I execute it as my free and voluntary act for the purposes therein expressed, and that I am of the age of majority or otherwise legally empowered to make a will, and under no constraint or under influence.

_____

NAME OF PERSON SIGNING WILL

On this _____ *day of*
_____*, 201__,*
_____ *declared to us, the
undersigned, that this instrument consisting of 3
pages was his will and requested us to act as
witnesses to it. He thereupon signed this will in our
presence, all of us being present at the same time.
We now, at his request, in his presence, and in the
presence of each other, subscribe our names as
witnesses and declare we understand this to be his
will, and that to the best of our knowledge the
testator is of the age of majority, or is otherwise
legally empowered to make a will, and is not acting
under duress, menace, fraud or misrepresentation
and is under no constraint or undue influence*

*We declare under penalty of perjury under the laws
of the State of California, that the foregoing is true
and correct.*

*Executed
at*_____,
on this _____ *day of* _____, *201___.*

WITNESSES #1

_____

residing at

WITNESS #2:

residing at

All of the necessary components for an effective will are in represented in the template you've just read, but you may have noticed that they're shrouded in a seeming impenetrable veil of "legalese." Let me translate to English for you.

FIRST: This part is just identifying your kin. Your spouse and children's names go here.

SECOND and **_THIRD_**: These parts identify and empower the "executor of the will." This is the person who has the often-unpleasant duty of distributing your possessions after your death.

The problem is that this a heavy burden to ask a person to bear, so you'd think the people creating the will would make sure this person is fully aware of what is expected of them, but you'd be wrong. I've seen it countless times – this family member or friend is in the midst of an emotional meltdown over their loss and, suddenly, they've got this huge job to do. I'm sure a heads-up would have been appreciated in those situations. But you're better than that – you'd never do that to someone you love, right?

The solution is simple: while you're drafting

RANDOM FACT: THE MOST ACCURATE WAY TO DETERMINE THE AGE OF A BEAR IS TO COUNT THE RINGS IN A CROSS SECTION OF ITS TOOTH ROOT UNDER A MICROSCOPE.

your will, call up the person you'd like to execute your will and talk to them about it. Let them know what would be expected of them, and then ask them to do this favor for you. Tell them that you would only ask them because you love and respect them. Acknowledge that what you're asking for is, indeed, a heavy burden to bear. Also, be willing to take on the same burden for this same loved one, should you survive them.

In many states, if your estate—the sum total of all of your assets—is valued at more than the $150,000, that estate may be probated.[33] Probate is the legal proceeding that is used to "wrap up" your legal and financial affairs after your death. The process can take at least eight months and sometimes as long as several years.

Probate can be a complex and expensive process. First, the executor you named must file a petition with the appropriate court to execute your estate. The will is also filed with the petition, and notices are sent to the heirs and/or relatives to let them know when the hearing will be held. If there are objections to the petition, or if the validity of the will is contested, the hearing will be used to resolve any problems that have arisen. In some cases this may mean that the validity of the will is not upheld,

---

[33] Be sure to check the probate laws in your state. I've chosen to focus on California because that's where my son—with whom I consulted with for this chapter--went to law school.

or that some person other than the original petitioner is chosen to administer the estate. In most cases, however, there is no objection and the petition is granted. The executor then makes an inventory of the estate's assets, locates creditors, pays bills, files tax returns, and manages the estate assets. When all of the duties of the executor are completed, another petition is filed with the court asking that the estate be distributed to the heirs. If this petition is granted, the estate administration is completed by distributing the assets to the heirs and filing final tax returns.

See what I'm talking about here? Being the executor of your will is like being the CEO of *You, Inc*. Choose carefully, request honestly.

Moving on.

FOURTH: This part spells out who you want all your stuff to go to and who's next on the list if the first people you select don't outlive you. This template has all possessions and property going to the spouse, but you can break it down item-by-item to spell out who gets what if you would like. That can get pretty complicated, so it's best to hire an estate lawyer to help you, should you choose that route.

FIFTH: This part assumes you're leaving all property and possessions to your spouse. If you got specific in *FOURTH*, then this part will change, too.

SIXTH: This part spells out what to do in the case of an heir contesting the will. The one in this template is a bit harsh – it says that if anyone contests any part of it, their share will be the same as if they had died before the person who wrote this will. Ouch.

There's a lot more this chapter could cover, but it has at least touched on the basics. For more detailed information, check out the links at the back of the book.

For information specific to your situation, be sure to contact your lawyer. If you don't have a lawyer, ask your friends for recommendations. If you can't afford a lawyer, check with a nearby law school. Many of them hold law clinics, where lawyers will help address your issues for free.

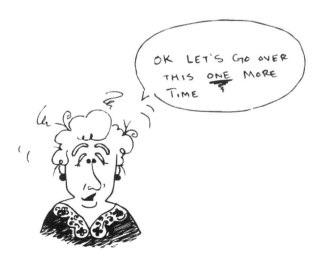

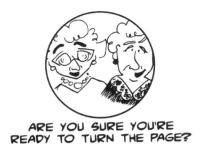

THE TALKING POINTS

Before moving on to the next chapter, be sure to cover these points in your follow-up conversation:

- If you have more than $25 is assets, you need to have a will. (That goes for everyone, regardless of age). Having a will is the responsible and compassionate thing to do.
- The best thing to do is to talk to a lawyer, but you should do your homework to save on billable hours. Take a look at the requirements for your state.
- Probate can be a nasty process. What can you do to avoid having to have your loved ones deal with it?
- Who do you trust to be the executor of your will? How will you approach the subject of being your executor with them? When are you going to talk to them?
- Don't play "executor yo-yo". One you've named an executor, stick with them. It gets really complicated if you don't.

- Make sure your will is up-to-date and bearing the name of your executor.
- Only have *one* version of your will in circulation.

HEART

10 THE PLEDGE TO AGE BRAVELY

I had a blog once; it lasted two days. I really wanted to have a forum where people could get together and talk openly and honestly about the difficulties in preparing for the final stage of life, but the first person to jump in also jumped on my case pretty hard. "How can *anyone* possibly plan for what's going to happen to them?" she exclaimed. I could tell she was dealing with a lot of pain and frustration.

After I began a dialogue with her, I learned that she had a relative who had once slapped her in the face. (Ordinarily, I'd chuckle at the way life works out sometimes, but this woman's heart-breaking response held even my sordid sense of humor in check.) The woman said she was only trying to explain to her weeping loved one—who suffered from dementia—where she could find her lost cat, but instead of gratitude, she got the back of a hand.

She misinterpreted what I was trying to say, taking it to mean that people can plan for everything. The truth is you can't – there is absolutely no way to predict what an patient suffering from dementia or Alzheimer's will do from one day to the next. However, you can *prepare* for anything. I'm not playing word games here – with a solid plan for dealing with the obstacles of aging, your elderly parent can be assured that they and their family will not be caught by surprise. I call this the "The Pledge to Age Bravely."

In my "day job" as a nurse practitioner on 24-hour call for multiple nursing homes, I see it every day – families in full panic mode because no one had a plan for dealing with an elder parent's health situation, and before everyone knew it, there it was – disaster staring them right in the face.

Most of the major events in adulthood are the product of a plan. Except in certain situations— usually those involving some measure of alcohol, the occurrence of which disproportionately transpires in the state of Nevada—you put some thought into your wedding and family planning. I'll bet you didn't buy your house on a whim. You didn't walk by and think "Sure, why the hell not?" Similarly, that car in your driveway isn't there because you were bored one day. So, why don't we apply the same degree of thoughtfulness to aging?

Part of the reason for this is societal. We, as a society, emphasize education from childhood to young adulthood, but then, for some reason that I fail to grasp, this emphasis disappears. We leave older adults to fend for themselves. "Oh, they'll figure it out." No, actually, they won't. I bear witness to this terrible truth every day.

The first step to taking the pledge is embracing the "Capital T" Truth: *There is no miracle cure for aging.* We get older, and then we die. There is absolutely, positively nothing you can do about it, and hiding from this fact is just makes the situation so much worse.

So, now that we've accepted this Truth, let's take a look at how to create an action plan:

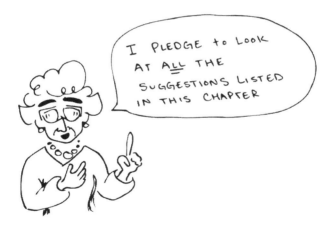

I PLEDGE to LooK AT ALL THE SUGGESTIONS LISTED IN THIS CHAPTER

RANDOM FACT: THE SMELL OF YOUNG WINE IS CALLED AN "AROMA" WHILE A MATURE WINE OFFERS A MORE SUBTLE "BOUQUET."

TEN THINGS TO A SENIOR NEEDS TO CONSIDER BEFORE TAKING THE PLEDGE

1. Change and challenges are inherent parts of aging. What you did and how you did things will not stay the same as you grow older.
2. Your relationship with your kids has changed; your job as their parent is over. Your kids are adults, so treat them accordingly.
3. This is uncharted territory for you. You've never been elderly before, so don't be afraid to say "I don't know." Nobody expects you to have all the answers.
4. You will most likely need some degree of assistance in your day-to-day, anywhere from basic activities of daily living (ADLs) to total care.
5. Your current living arrangements may not always accommodate your needs.
6. How you grow old is up to you. If you *choose* not to make plans, the consequences are a direct result of that choice.
7. Making plans safeguards your independence even while in the state of dependence. In other words, if you claim your right to "call the shots," you will never lose it.
8. Because "no man is an island," plans need to be shared. Once you complete the Pledge, talk to your family about it. They can only help you carry out your wishes if they know about them.

9. At this stage in life, *legacy* becomes an important consideration. When making decisions, ask yourself, "How will this affect how I am remembered?"

10. Once you've made these decision, you must create a plan and *set a deadline* to complete the tasks I've assigned. Put it on your calendar!

THE PLEDGE TO AGE BRAVELY

I _____, do hereby set in motion my plan to "Age Bravely." I realize that this is not a legally binding document, but it is to be considered an important demonstration of my purposed aging plan.

PART 1: *If I have not had the opportunity to be involved with an elder's life to witness their challenges first hand, I pledge to observe institutionalized elders. I understand that this assignment is meant for me to observe different disease processes that can affect one's independence and to witness firsthand just how these processes may affect living arrangements. The purpose of these observation exercises is to help me make decisions regarding my own care, in the event that similar physical/ medical challenges affect my own life.*

- *I understand that a minimum of two visits will be required to obtain a full impression.*
- *I will record my impressions of each facility in order to develop a solid understanding of what I want.*
- *I understand that this plan is not final and that regular reviews and modifications will be ongoing.*

- *I understand there is "leg work" involved with establishing a plan.*
- *I will contact and observe at least two nursing homes, two assisted living residencies, and two group homes.*

* * * * *

PART 2: THE "LEGWORK"

NURSING HOME #1: *I visited*

_____,

on _____, *20___.*

My Impressions:

_____

_____

_____

_____

_____

NURSING HOME #2: *I visited*

_____,

on _____, *20___.*

My Impressions:

_____

_____

_____

_____

_____

ASSISTED LIVING RESIDENCY #1*: I visited*

_____,

on _____, *20___.*

My Impressions:

_____

_____

_____

_____

_____

ASSISTED LIVING RESIDENCY #2*: I visited*

_____,

on _____, *20___.*

My Impressions:

_____

_____

_____

_____

_____

GROUP HOME #1: *I visited*

_____,

on _____, *20___.*

My Impressions:

_____

_____

_____

_____

_____

GROUP HOME #2: *I visited*

_____,

on _____, *20___.*

My Impressions:

_____

_____

_____

_____

_____

PART 3: *I recognize that knowledge is power, and I do seek to be the master of my own fate; I will empower myself through education. I will use the resources listed in the back of this book to research the following important items:*

- **The three leading forms of cancer:**

    1) _____

    Mortality Rate:

    _____

    Treatment Options:

    _____

    _____

2) _____

Mortality Rate: _____

Treatment Options:

_____

_____

3) _____

Mortality Rate:

_____

Treatment Options:

_____

_____

• **The three major debilitating disease processes most common in the following age groups:**

   o **50-60s:**

      1.) _____

      2.) _____

      3.) _____

○ *60-70:*

    1.) _____

    2.) _____

    3.) _____

○ *70-80:*

    1.) _____

    2.) _____

    3.) _____

○ *80 up :*

    1.) _____

    2.) _____

    3.) _____

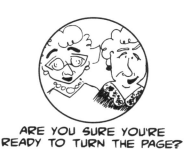

ARE YOU SURE YOU'RE
READY TO TURN THE PAGE?

THE TALKING POINTS

You've just covered some weighty stuff in this chapter. Aging bravely is a heavy burden to bear, but they don't have to do it alone. These are some of the things you two should talk about after taking the Pledge to Age Bravely:

- Think about the memories you have of the elders in your life? What did you admire about them? What irritated you about them? Did anything horrify you about them?
- What does "legacy" mean to you? What do you want your legacy to be?
- What can we do to make sure you have the legacy you want?
- What do you think of the Pledge to Age Bravely? Would you be willing to make that commitment?
- How could we maintain your independence even when you make the transition to a state of dependence?
- Now that the complicated stuff has been addressed, considered and outlined, your

parent really needs to go on and live their life to the fullest. There's a beach chair with their name on it, now they need to go find it!

11 THE FINAL CHAPTER

If I were forced to describe the aim of this book with a single word, that word would have to be *control*.[34] It seems like from the time we take our very first breath to the time we take our very last, life—that little thing in the middle—is one constant struggle for control. We gain it, we lose it, and sometimes we have to compromise our control, but those who *age bravely* never give up that fight.

If your parent has taken this book to heart, then by now they've taken all the necessary steps to ensure they live the rest of your days on their own terms – they have re-taken control of their lives. But we're not finished yet. There's just one last thing

---

[34] Distilling something complicated down to a single word is a great way to come to understand it. For instance, if you're having an argument with a loved one, try taking a moment and have both of you say what's really bothering you in one word. Sometimes too many words can just get in the way of what you're really trying to say.

they need to do: plan for the final chapter.

Yes, I'm talking about *death*.

I know, I know; you're probably terrified of that word, but you shouldn't be. Our culture has ingrained in us this certainty that death means a total loss of control of your life, but I don't buy it— not for a second.

Don't get me wrong – I'm not arguing that you have any sort of control over what happens to you after you die. (That's left up to someone with more credentials than me.) I'm saying that you have the power to control the impact of your death on those you love. If you do this right, you'll never actually die.

The key to this death-defying feat is actually fairly simple. It's a concept you may even have heard of: *legacy*.

Webster's defines *legacy* as "something transmitted by or received from an ancestor or predecessor or from the past." We often think of this as money or property, i.e. "legacy funds," but there's another meaning—one which pertains to something much more valuable. Legacy is the term we use to describe how you will be remembered by those you leave behind.

An important note before we move on to the meat of this chapter: I'm not going to be offering advice on how to live your life in a way that assures you will be remembered well. There are plenty of books on this topic, several of which were written by well-respected authors.[35] I want to address something that our culturally ingrained fear of death so often prevents us from doing – planning for our deaths.

How does planning for your death affect your legacy? Excellent question. Let's say you somehow managed to live your life in such a way that you're a shoe-in for beatification.[36] Good for you! Let's also say you died without leaving your family a plan for what to do with your body. Well, now instead of having the time to properly grieve the passing of a loved one, they have to plan and pay for your funeral, with only their imaginations to figure out what you would have wanted in this situation. Their memory of you is tarnished because of this one selfish act. Get it now?

---

[35] Muhammad, Moses, and Stephen R. Covey, just to name a few.

[36] "A recognition accorded by the Catholic Church of a dead person's entrance into Heaven and capacity to intercede on behalf of individuals who pray in his or her name (intercession of saints)."

This chapter will walk you through the process of planning your final chapter. If you get this right, you've assured your control of your life long after you are gone. In your own little way, you will have triumphed over death. (Beat that, Stephen R. Covey!)

Call me a big meanie, but when I'm about to address a serious issue with one of my patients, I like to give them a real-life horror story or two first to illustrate what could happen if they don't take the advice I'm about to give them. (I find this helps to cement my point.) So, here are yours:

This is a story of loose ends.

The other day I was taking a new patient's medical history, and when I got to the part of the interview in which I ask if the patient has a living will or advance directive, he said "no." (What a shocker!) I then set off on my usual rant about the importance of protecting one's health rights and wishes. He listened and acted, and I'm proud of him.

But here's the thing that gets me – he shouldn't have needed me to hit him over the head with the facts before he would face them. He'd seen what happens first-hand if you don't plan ahead, because he had already had to deal with the death of *his own mother*.

This patient's mother had been widowed for about five years when she found someone with whom she wanted to spend the rest of her days. They got married, and they were happy for five years. Then, the gentleman died. She grieved for a few more years before she herself died. During the last few years of her life, she and my patient, the eldest of twelve children, had a couple of informal discussions about her last wishes. During one of these chats, he asked a really good question – "Do you want to be buried with your first or second husband?" She thought about it and decided to be buried with the second. However, they never committed her wishes to paper.

After she passed, the twelve children came together to discuss burial plans. My patient told his siblings about the conversations he'd had with their mother and how she'd told him she wanted to be buried with her second husband. This offended several of his siblings, as their father was her first husband. He argued that it wasn't their choice to

RANDOM FACT: BRISK WALKING HELPS REDUCE BODY FAT, LOWER BLOOD PRESSURE, AND INCREASE HIGH-DENSITY LIPOPROTEIN.

make – it's what *she* had wanted that was important. After much debate, they took a vote. She came within two votes of being buried with the wrong man.

If she had followed the advice in this chapter, her eternal resting place wouldn't have come down to a slim majority of votes.

One more thing to consider before moving on from this sad tale – the mother's legacy was, in the eyes of the children who lost the vote, forever tarnished. While they may have resented her somewhat for instructing them to bury them with a man who was not their father, they ultimately would have respected her wishes. However, by not leaving them instructions, those children see her as pitting them against their siblings in a battle to do what they thought was best for her. In fact, a number of those siblings won't talk to each other to this day. They are a family no more. Her failure to act destroyed in days what she had worked decades to create.

Ready for one more?

A widowed gentleman suffering from the slow degeneration of Alzheimer's took up what would become a decade of lonely residence in a nursing home.

Despite being estranged from his father for many years, his son was still listed as "next of kin." No one had been appointed power of attorney before the man died. Thus, the son, who had tried so hard to forget about his father, got a phone call from a desperate nursing home administrator looking for someone to instruct her as to what to do with the body. You can imagine his surprise.

The son, not having a clue as to what his father would have wanted, ordered a cremation and went about setting up a memorial for the man.

It was at the memorial where his horrified aunt, the deceased's sister, confronted him. "Didn't you remember how terrified your father was of fire?" she demanded. "Now you've damned him to eternal hellfire! How could you be so cruel?"

The young man could only shake his head and walk away, forever resenting the man who raised him.

I think I've made my point. Let's move on to the part where I tell you how to avoid tragedies like these.

So, I'm dead. Now what?

The first thing you have to do is decide what you want done with your body after you're gone. No matter what you believe spiritually, you probably won't need it anymore, and you just can't leave it lying about. There are several options available to you, and each one has its pros and cons. Let's take a look.

Organ Donation. Look, you've no longer got a use for your organs anymore, so why not use the occasion of your death as an opportunity to give a stranger the greatest gift of all – a second chance at life?[37]

Some things to consider:[38]

- Another name is added to the national transplant waiting list every 12 minutes.
- On average, 18 people die every day from the lack of available organs for transplant.

---

[37] Get the facts here: http://www.organdonor.gov/whydonate/facts.html

[38] Get more facts and find out how to become an organ donor here: http://www.americantransplantfoundation.org/about-transplant/facts-and-myths/

- One organ donor can save up to eight lives. The same donor can also save or improve the lives of up to 50 people by donating tissues and eyes.
- All major religions support organ donation.
- In many states, all you have to do to become an organ donor is to go to your local DMV and tell them you want to be a donor. They will update your license to indicate your status.

I urge you to consider becoming an organ donor. If you think about it, there are absolutely no downsides to becoming one. Nobody's going to take your organs until you're done using them (that would be very rude), and it's quite possible that by giving this gift, a physical part of you will exist long after you are gone.

Organ donation is a wonderful thing, but still leaves a question – what do you do with the rest of the body?

Cremation. Genesis 3:19: "In the sweat of thy face shalt thou eat bread, till thou return unto the ground; for out of it wast thou taken: for dust thou art, and unto dust shalt thou return."

Cremation is "the use of high-temperature burning, vaporization, and oxidation to reduce dead animal bodies, including human ones, to basic chemical compounds, such as gases and mineral fragments."[39]

While public opinions still steer more towards traditional burial, there are several reasons why you should consider this option. Let's take a look at a few:[40]

- Cost: On average, cremation is one-third the cost of burial. Have you seen the costs associated with traditional burials? It's staggering. (We'll get into that later.)
- Convenience: Migration to retirement locations is increasing, and the further away seniors move from their old homes, the less likely they are to have loved ones nearby to visit their grave.
- Simplicity: With a direct cremation, your loved ones will never need to go to a funeral home. All paperwork can be handled from home. (Makes it easier for them to focus on dealing with their grief.)
- Environmentally responsible: The embalming fluid used in traditional

---

[39] From Wikipedia

[40] Provided by the Cremation Association of North America.

burials has been known to leach into groundwater. Also, many environmentally conscious people are choosing cremation because they feel "land should be left for the living," meaning with land being in shorter supply, it can be put to better use than burying the dead.

- Bonding experience: The act of spreading the ashes is an ideal opportunity to bring your family closer together. Pick a spot you that meant a lot to you and have your family gather there. (Note: there is no law saying the ashes have to be spread. Mausoleums and even mantles are popular options.)

- The best part: there's no rush to spread your ashes. Just have your family pick the time that's most convenient for everyone so they can experience the celebration of your life in a stress-free way.

Cremation is certainly an option to consider, but there are a couple of downsides to bear in mind:

- Burning bodies that have been embalmed in treated wood caskets releases dioxin, hydrochloric acid, hydrofluoric acid, sulfur dioxide, mercury (from dental work) and carbon dioxide into the air. Therefore, it's best not to cremate bodies prepared for traditional burial.

- It takes a lot of fossil fuel energy to burn a human body. If you were able to harness the energy from cremations done in a single year in the United States and you'd have enough to travel to the moon and back 83 times.

Traditional burial. Well, there's really not too much to say about traditional burial. It's traditional. I'd wager that you've been to at least one, so you probably know what it entails. Therefore, I'll use this space to bring up a few things about traditional burial that the funeral industry doesn't like to mention.

- According to AARP, funeral and burial costs can easily reach as much as $10,000.
- The embalming involves removing all bodily fluids and gasses and replacing blood with a formaldehyde-based solution for preserving and disinfecting. The World Health Organization classifies formaldehyde as a carcinogen. As of 2010,

RANDOM FACT: U.S. CHOCOLATE MANUFACTURERS USE ABOUT 35 MILLION POUNDS OF WHOLE MILK EVERY DAY TO MAKE MILK CHOCOLATE.

formaldehyde is banned in the European Union because of its carcinogenic effects.
- To keep up with American demand, approximately 30 million board feet (71,000 meters³) of casket wood is felled every year.
- The amount of steel used in caskets and vaults yearly in North America is equivalent to the amount used in the Golden Gate Bridge.

That being said, if you want a traditional burial, have one! There's something to be said for tradition. When a spouse dies and is buried, the widower usually wants to be buried beside their mate. A shared plot strikes me as one of the most beautiful displays of affection I've ever seen.

While this is the most expensive of the options we're covering, it doesn't have to be outrageously expensive – it's a buyer's market, so shop for the best deal. For example, did you know Costco sells caskets? Yes, *that* Costco. Other on- line "casket shops" can save you thousands. The funeral home will not care (by law!).

"Green" Burial (aka "Natural Burial"). This is an ancient concept that is coming back in a big way as our culture becomes more concerned about the environment. Green burial is quite simply burying the dead in a manner that does not inhibit decomposition, but allows the body to recycle naturally.

The problem many people have with embalming, in addition to the carcinogenic properties discussed above, is that it destroys the microbial decomposers that break the body down. In essence, you've been mummified for all eternity, and some people think that's just creepy.

Further, according to the Green Burial Council, this burial method also creates "minimal environmental impact that furthers legitimate ecological aims such as the conservation of natural resources, reduction of carbon emissions, protection of worker health, and the restoration and/or preservation of habitat."

I can't think of any downsides associated with this method, so here are a couple more selling points:

- You have more location options available. In addition to cemeteries, natural burials can take place on private land in most states.

- This method is already the standard for both Judaism and Islam.
- Instead of an expensive coffin, often constructed of exotic woods and with environmentally harmful production methods, popular burial containers include wicker baskets, shrouds and favorite blankets.

Okay. Now what?

Now it's time to do the responsible and compassionate thing and plan your funeral. Pre-planning and pre-paying for your funeral relieves your loved ones of the need to go through a complex (and often unpleasant) process at a time when they should be grieving your passing.

Notice I mentioned pre-paying just then? Depending on your preferred burial method, this can be a very expensive ordeal. Why would you want to force that financial burden on the people you leave behind? Remember your legacy here. No one wants to be remembered as the parsimonious jerk that couldn't chip in for his own funeral. In the

---

RANDOM FACT: IN 1923, MARK SENNETT, HARRY CHANDLER, AND THE LOS ANGELES TIMES PUT UP THE "HOLLYWOODLAND" (LATER SHORTENED TO "HOLLYWOOD") SIGN TO PUBLICIZE A REAL ESTATE DEVELOPMENT.

event you are, in fact, a cheapskate, here's a bit of good news: you may actually save a lot of money by pre-paying.

I'm not talking necessarily about pre-purchasing your funeral services from a vendor. In fact, this may be a bad idea. According to AARP, funeral homes, particularly those that have changed hands, do not always honor prepaid contracts or the agreed-upon prices.

What I *am* advising is that you set up a savings account specifically for burial expenses. Put a set amount of money into that account every month. By the time you need to use it, it should cover the majority of your expenses, and your family won't have to eat ramen noodles for the next year.

Planning Your Going Away Party

Who was the killjoy who made the hard and steadfast rule that funerals have to be these melancholy events that people loathe attending? Don't get me wrong – I'm not saying your funeral should be a raging kegger (although that might be fun), I'm merely pointing out there *are no rules* for this sort of thing. If you want your funeral to be traditional, go for it. If you want to make your funeral as unique as you were, there's nobody saying you can't. Whether you want people wearing party hats and singing "Louie, Louie" or quiet mourners singing "Amazing Grace," it's up to you. (We yuppies are changing everything.)

The key to getting this event the way your loved one wants it is just like that of the advance directive and living will we talked about earlier – spell out what you want! Luckily, we live in the online age and there are a lot of helpful websites out there to assist you guys.[41]

This is a list of things to consider when planning your event. After you've given these options some thought, you might want to fill out this form I've provided and give a copy to the person you've appointed power of attorney

- **Visitation: the place to pay your respects**
  - ○ Do you want one?
  - ○ Where do you want it to be? In a funeral home? What about outdoors with a beautiful backdrop? Set the tone.
  - ○ What do you want displayed? Photos, personal items, etc.

---

[41] In doing research for this chapter, I came across a great website called mywonderfullife.com. This site walks you step-by-step through planning just the funeral you want and gives you the ability to send your plan to loved ones. It is a commercial site, so they want you to buy stuff, but this service is free.

- Do you want music? Choose music that means something to you. It doesn't have to be appropriate for the environment; it's the soundtrack of your life.
- **Memorial**
  - Do you want one?
  - Eulogy: Appoint someone early. Nobody likes making a speech on the fly. You should also feel free to make suggestions.
  - Program: Design according to your taste: traditional, modern, or minimalistic? Content: Pictures Hymns? Poems? Quotes?
  - Consider making a video or writing a letter to be shared at the event.
- **Contributions**
  - In lieu of flowers, attendees can donate to charities that were important to you.
- **Obituary**
  - Where would you like it to be published? What would you like it to say?
  - These are the things typically included: date/place of birth, occupation, family members, and something interesting about you.
- **Pallbearers**
  - If you're going to have a casket, you'll need pallbearers. This is also a way to

honor those you loved. Let those you
choose know ahead of time.
- **Symbolic goodbyes?**
  - ○ Many interesting traditions: sprinkling
    dirt, laying roses, planting trees, flying
    kites, releasing balloons, butterflies, etc.
    Get creative!

Here's a nice little touch: Why not set aside a
little money for something special for your
immediate family to do after your memorial or
burial? I would suggest a private memorial dinner
somewhere or maybe a little getaway for your kids
(perhaps to spread your ashes along the way).
Here's an example: my mother-in-law loved the
Chinese buffet near her house. She wanted to make
sure we were all eating during this time of grief, so
she instructed the family to go there after paying
our respects. We did, and it was nice.

The Final Step

After your parent dies, there are a couple of
immediate issues that need to be resolved. The first
is to remove the body. If they died in a nursing
home, the facility will have a procedure for that.
But what about if they died at home? Well, it

varies.[42]

If your parent was enrolled in a hospice program (highly recommended), the paperwork for the medical examiner's office was pre-filed. All that needs to be done is for the hospice nurse to pronounce the death for the death certificate. After that, the hospice office will notify the funeral home, and the funeral home will come to take the body away.

If they were not on hospice, the procedure will vary by state. My best advice is to call 911 and unlock the front door; Paramedics and police will respond. If your parent had a DNR, make sure the family produces it upon arrival. The paramedics will honor it and won't try to perform CPR. (FYI: The paramedics will ignore an advance directive – that only concerns doctors and the care of terminal patients.) Just so you know, the police and medical examiner will investigate the scene and instruct you further.

Once that part is finished, the notification process begins. I would start with immediate family. If your parent was sick for a while, they've been

---

[42] For detailed instructions, check out Elder Care Team: http://www.eldercareteam.com/public/757print.cfm

anticipating this call. (Make sure it's a call. Texting this kind of news is *really* inappropriate.) After the funeral, you will need to get a death certificate before the next round of notifications.[43] Once you have that, you will need to cancel credit cards, bank accounts[44], insurance and social security. Be sure to notify the IRS, too. They will try to collect taxes otherwise.

I've included a handy "Important Personal Information" at the back of the book. Simply have your parent fill in all of their financial information (bank account numbers, 401K info, locations of safety deposit boxes, etc.) to help the executor expedite the closing of all of their accounts.

---

[43] The procedure for obtaining a death certificate varies slightly by state. Here's a link to California's application process through the Department of Public Health: http://www.cdph.ca.gov/certlic/birthdeathmar/pages/certifiedcopiesofbirthdeathrecords.aspx

[44] This is more complex at some banks than at others. Ask ahead for the procedure.

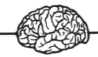

DID YOU KNOW?

Hospice is a wonderful and FREE Medicare service for the terminally ill.

Includes a Hospice Team: nurses, nursing aids, social workers and a staff chaplain who travel to your home or care facility.

100% of the expense of medicines, equipment and products is covered by Medicare.

Respite Care is available to give the family a break from the pressure, including in-patient care at a temporary facility.

They have 24/7 phone support available during care and then 14 months of bereavement support for the family afterward.

In Conclusion

Here's one of my husband's favorite corny jokes: "What does it mean when the pastor says 'In conclusion'? Absolutely nothing." Well, I didn't go to seminary, so this really is the end.

But before I go, I just want to mention two more things:

1. I am *so* very proud of you. Confronting the issues we discussed in this book can be really unpleasant. Now that you've dealt with them, you've got nothing left to really worry about. Focus on living your life to the maximum. Age bravely!
2. Don't skimp on the hugs. Life is tragically short. Don't miss the opportunity to show people how much they mean to you.

Remember, we're in this together. If you need me, reach out.

Facebook.com/AgingBravely

My Funeral Details

<u>My Body</u>

I want to be: □ Traditionally Buried □ Naturally Buried □ Cremated

How, Where, and Special Instructions:

_____

_____

_____

_____

_____

_____

I want to a: □ Headstone □ Memorial □ N/A

<u>Visitation</u>

I want this: □ Yes □ No

Location: _____

Items to Display:

_____

_____

_____

Music to Be Played:

_____

_____

_____

Special Instructions:

_____

_____

Memorial

I want this: ☐ Yes ☐ No

Location: _____

Eulogy: ☐ Yes ☐ No

Eulogist:

_____

Eulogy Suggestions:

_____

_____

_____

Music to Be Played:

_____

_____

_____

Passages and/or Poems to Be Read:

_____

_____

_____

Program Style:

_____

Program Content:

_____

_____

Contributions

I want this: ☐ Yes ☐ No

Charity or Cause:

_____

Obituary

I want this: ☐ Yes ☐ No

Where to Publish:

_____

What to Say:

_____

_____

_____

_____

_____

_____

Pallbearers

I want this: ☐ Yes ☐ No

Names:

_____

_____

_____

Symbolic Goodbyes

I want this: ☐ Yes ☐ No

Suggestions:

_____

_____

Further Instructions

_____

_____

_____

_____

_____

_____

_____

_____

_____

_____

IMPORTANT PERSONAL INFORMATION

Your executor needs your help closing out your accounts after you have passed on. Be sure to complete this list of critical items and make sure they have a copy.

1. Safety Deposit Boxes
    a. Location: _____
    b. Keys are: _____
2. Personal Safes
    a. Location: _____
    b. Keys/Combination:

    _____
    _____

3. Bank Accounts
    a. Bank Names:

    _____
    _____

    b. Account Numbers:

    _____
    _____
    _____

4. 401K: _____
5. Passwords to Important Websites:

    _____
    _____

RESOURCES

BOOKS

Cohen, Gene D. *The Creative Age: Awakening Human Potential in the Second Half of Life*. New York: Quill, 2000. Paperback.

Colvin Rhodes, Linda. *The Complete Idiot's Guide to Caring for Aging Parents*. Indianapolis: Alpha Books, 2001. Paperback.

Dugan, Elizabeth. *The Driving Dilemma: The Complete Resource Guide for Older Drivers and Their Families*. New York: William Morrow Paperbacks, 2006. Paperback.

Henry, Stella Mora. *The Eldercare Handbook: Difficult Choices, Compassionate Solutions*. New York: Collins, 2006. Paperback.

Loverde, Joy. *The Complete Eldercare Planner:*

Where to Start, Which Questions to Ask, and How to Find Help. New York: Three Rivers Press, 2009. Paperback.

Solie, David. *How to Say it to Seniors: Closing the Communication Gap with our Elders*. New York: Prentice Hall Press, 2004. Paperback.

Taylor, Dan. *The Parent Care Conversation: Six Strategies for Dealing with the Emotional and Financial Challenges of Aging Parents*. New York: Penguin Books, 2006. Paperback.

Thomas, William H. *What Are Old People For?* Acton: VanderWyk Burnham, 2007. Paperback.

ONLINE RESOURCES

Chapter 1

"New Insight Into the Fear of Aging"
http://www.huffingtonpost.com/2012/06/19/new-insight-into-the-fear-of-aging_n_1607305.html

"Learning to Love Growing Old"
http://www.psychologytoday.com/articles/199409/learning-love-growing-old

"Your Aging Parents Are Now Senior Citizens: How to Talk About the Future"
http://www.talk-early-talk-often.com

"How to Talk to the Elderly About Tough Family Issues"
http://www.caring.com/articles/talking-to-elderly-parents

"Connecting People Caring for Elderly Parents"
http://www.agingcare.com

Chapter 2
"Understanding Advance Directives"

http://www.caringinfo.org/files/public/brochures/
Understanding_Advance_Directives.pdf

"Why Do We Avoid Advance Directives?"
http://newoldage.blogs.nytimes.com/2009/04/20/
why-do-we-avoid-advance-directives/

 "Download Your State's Advance Directive"
http://www.caringinfo.org/i4a/pages/index.cfm?
pageid=3289

Chapter 3
"What is Dementia?"
http://www.alz.org/what-is-dementia.asp

"Dementia: Causes, Symptoms, Test, Treatment,
Prevention"
http://www.dementia.org

"Alzheimer's Association"
http://www.alz.org

"Alzheimer's Foundation of America"
http://www.alzfdn.org

 Chapter 4
 "What You Should Know About DNR Orders"

https://www.ohiobar.org/ForPublic/Resources/
LawYouCanUse/Pages/LawYouCanUse-299.aspx

"Understanding CPR and DNR Orders"
http://www.cancer.net/coping/end-life-care/
understanding-cpr-and-dnr-orders

"Understanding Living Wills and DNR Orders"
http://patientsafetyauthority.org/ADVISORIES/
AdvisoryLibrary/2008/Dec5(4)/Pages/111.aspx

Chapter 5

"Artificial Nutrition: Feeding Tubes and IVs at the
End of Life"
http://dying.about.com/od/lifesupport/a/
artificialfeed

"Common Questions and Answers About Artificial
Nutrition and Hydration"
http://www.baylorhealth.com/
SiteCollectionDocuments/Documents_BHCS/
BHCS_Patient%20Info_DocumentsForms/
ArtificialNutritionHydration_rev7.pdf

Chapter 6

"Making Peace with Our Elderly Parents"
http://www.mentalhelp.net/poc/view_doc.php?

type=docid=36378

"Caring for Elderly Parents"
http://www.aplaceformom.com/senior-care-resources/articles/caring-for-elderly-parentsm

"How to Handle an Elderly Parent's Bad Behavior"
http://www.agingcare.com/Articles/bad-behavior-by-elderly-parents-138673.htm

Chapter 7
"Aging Parents Moving In"
http://www.aarp.org/home-family/caregiving/info-06-2012/afford-aging-parents-moving-in.html

"Assisted Living Source"
http://www. assistedlivingsource.com

"Senior Resource: Shared Housing for Seniors"
http://www.seniorresource.com/shared.htm

"Medicare and You: Getting Started"
http://www.aarp.org/health/medicare-insurance/info-01-2011/understanding_medicare_a_boomers_guide.html

"The Official U.S. Government Site for Medicare"

http://www.medicare.gov

Chapter 8
"Elderly Driving Statistics"
http://seniors.lovetoknow.com/
Elderly_Driving_Statistics

"Senior Driving 101"
http://www.caring.com/about-senior-driving

"Driver Improvement Courses For Seniors"
http://seniordriving.aaa.com/maintain-mobility-
independence/driver-improvement-courses-seniors

"A Contract to Stop Driving"
http://newoldage.blogs.nytimes.com/2011/11/30/a-
contract-to-stop-driving/

Chapter 9
"Understanding Wills"
http://www.azbar.org/workingwithlawyers/topics/
willsandtrusts

"Making a Simple Will"
http://www.calbar.ca.gov/Public/SimpleWill.aspx

"Will Requirements by State"

http://www.lawserver.com/will-requirements-by-state

Chapter 11
"My Wonderful Life: Your Own Funeral Planning Website"
http://www.mywonderfullife.com

"Funeral Planning Information and Tools"
http://www.thefuneralsite.com/ResourceCenters/

"FAQs Fiction" Green Burial
http://www.greenburialcouncil.org/faqs-fiction/

Random Facts
The "Random Facts" featured throughout the book are from facts.randomhistory.com

ABOUT THE AUTHOR

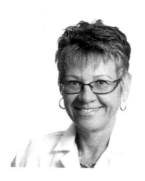

Dana was a stay-at-home mom in her 30s with three children when she decided to go back to school. After several years of juggling kids and textbooks, she was awarded a B.S. in Nursing from Texas Women's University.

After two decades of working in geriatrics, oncology, and hospice, she returned to school to earn her M.S. in Nursing. Now a nurse practitioner, Dana has renewed her geriatrics focus through clinical practice and a new avenue—advocacy.

Dana lives in Dallas, Texas, where she and her husband spend their time spoiling their first grandchild rotten.

THANKS FOR READING & "AGING BRAVELY"!

NOTES

Made in the USA
San Bernardino, CA
11 July 2013